Table of contents

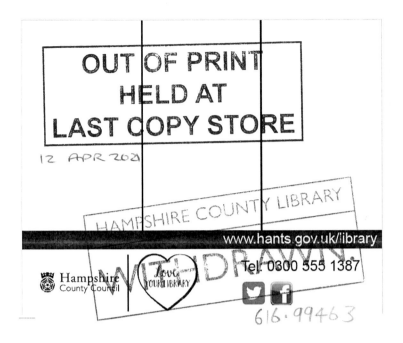
The story of my prostatectomy and
a rough guide for the prostate cancer journey

by

Giuseppe Enrico Bignardi

This book is published by
Grosvenor House Publishing Ltd
Link House
140 The Broadway, Tolworth, Surrey, KT6 7HT
www.grosvenorhousepublishing.co.uk

A CIP record for this book
is available from the British Library

ISBN 978-1-78623-064-5

Acknowledgments

First of all, I would like to thank my wonderful wife Margherita. Margherita is the best thing that has happened to me in my life and I would not have coped with the prostate cancer diagnosis so well without her. I am also very grateful to my urology surgeon for the great skill with which he performed my prostatectomy.

This book, however, is primarily dedicated to my two sons: Agostino and Giacomo. Now you know that your dad has prostate cancer, and that you are at increased risk of facing the same challenge. But there are many things that you can start doing now to reduce the risk. Above all, if you were diagnosed later in life with prostate cancer, or any other conditions, there are things you can do to maximise your chances of choosing the right treatment and to get the best possible outcomes.

The icon of a man, on the front cover was made by Freepik from www.flaticon.com.

Introduction

There are three sections in this book. "The story of my prostatectomy" is the story (so far) of my prostate cancer. "The story of my life" (limited to a few key events) follows, and it may help to put things in perspective: it may explain how I reacted and how I intend to fight my battle. After that, the "rough guide for prostatectomy patients" is a list of what we can do to help ourselves, ranging from how to choose our prostate cancer treatment up to how we can maximise our chances of response. This is a "rough" guide: not really a proper authoritative guide. Experts may write definitive guide books. I am no expert, I am a fellow traveller on the prostate cancer journey: all I have done is to reflect and search for answers. And all I can offer is a personal opinion and some sign posts to more authoritative sources. There is a key message in this book: we need to be "active" patients.

I hope other fellow travellers, on the same prostate cancer journey, may find the shared information useful. The book is also intended for the close male relatives of prostate cancer patients; they need to give some thought to their increased risk of prostate cancer, and start working on reducing it. They also need to consider whether they want to go for screening, and how they would manage the screening results.

The story of my prostatectomy

Sunday, 23 October 2016 (the day before)

The robotic prostatectomy is due tomorrow. Alarm clock set for 5am: shower and the last sachet of Vitaflo pre-load carbohydrates. Then off to the hospital.

Have I made the right treatment choice?

I accepted the proposed robotic prostatectomy because I felt I disliked surgery less than radiotherapy or androgen deprivation therapy. But, it is possible the prostate cancer has already extended beyond the capsule of the prostate or has spread to the lymph nodes. It is also possible that adjuvant or salvage radiotherapy will be proposed after the surgical procedure.

The thing is, the prostate cancer has not given me any trouble so far, it was an unexpected finding when I went to my GP and asked to check my testosterone levels (it seems all problems men have later in life are due to the "andropause" and testosterone supplementation might be the answer). The GP said I would need to do a PSA test as well, as he would not prescribe testosterone replacement if my PSA was abnormally high. In the end the testosterone was in the normal range but the PSA was quite high (21 ng/ml). The obvious thing to do was to ask for a repeat PSA test: surely it was a mistake in the lab. The second PSA was a bit better (15 ng/ml) but still quite high. I was told I would be mad if I refused to be investigated with prostatic biopsies. I am a

1

medical microbiologist: the only men with prostatic biopsies I see are those returning to hospital with post-biopsy sepsis. I tried to buy time, I pleaded for a multiparametric MRI: the MRI showed a lesion in the prostate. At that stage I was really trapped: I could not turn down the "offer" of prostatic biopsies, could I? The urologist also requested a bone scan, because the MRI had shown a possible lesion in the pelvic bones, though not typical of metastasis.

Thanks God the bone scan did not show evidence of metastases. The biopsies were transperineal (not the more common transrectal type) as this was thought to be a better way to reach the anterior part of my prostate, where my "lesion" was. The biopsies were done on 12 September under general anaesthesia. I left the hospital a few hours later with a big haematoma over the perineal and scrotal area, and pissing blood. Cold packs seemed to help to reduce the haematoma swelling and the gross haematuria stopped a few hours later, after I passed an obvious blood clot with my urine. Blood in the sperm continued for more than a month, but it looked like "old" blood.

I went to my outpatient appointment to discuss the histology result with the understanding that, despite my high PSA, I still had about a 50% chance of not having a prostate cancer. Surely, I did not have a prostate cancer: I am "only" 60 and very fit (gym five times a week), not overweight and I follow a good healthy Mediterranean diet (I am a British Italian, if it makes sense: I have both nationalities and I feel a bit of both). Also, I do not know of any male relatives who had prostate cancer. For years I have taken vitamin D supplements, which should reduce the risk of prostate cancer. And have I mentioned that for years I had taken a glass of pomegranate juice at dinner, having read it could reduce the risk of prostate cancer?

So, what will happen tomorrow? The surgeon has said he would like to do a lymph node dissection as well. It seems it could help, even if (I think) I am still categorised as "intermediate" risk (Gleason score 3+4, hopefully T2 stage but cannot be sure, PSA mean value 17 out of 4 tests). But what if the tumour is already extending outside the prostatic capsule (the histology report mentioned this might be the case on the left side) or has already spread to the lymph nodes? What if my surgeon says I need radiotherapy as well? I have a mild form of ulcerative colitis and this might be exacerbated by radiotherapy. And what about the other radiotherapy side-effects and long-term risks?

The discussion about my treatment options sounded a little bit like this: we are going to give you a "beating" (unavoidable side-effects from any of the treatment options) but you have a "choice". We can beat you with a wooden stick (prostatectomy) or with an iron bar (radiotherapy). But, if you choose the wooden stick because you think it is less painful, we still reserve the right to use the iron bar later. Should I have gone for a single beating with the iron bar?

I am a bit worried about tomorrow. I might be in the 5% group with more serious surgical side-effects. Will I really ever recover my continence? It feels to me I have run out of luck. I agreed to a PSA test because I was confident it would be normal. I asked for a repeat PSA test because surely the high result was attributable to sex the night before. I asked for an MRI because a normal result would have allowed me to refuse prostatic biopsies. I accepted prostatic biopsies knowing I still had a 50% chance of being clear. I have lost all the game rounds so far. Will I lose the next game? I am not a football fanatic, but I work in Sunderland, a city whose football team has often struggled at the bottom of the Premiership table. I know that when a football teams starts to lose games repeatedly, sometimes it never stops until you get relegated to a lower division. Will I lose my next game (surgery)? Will I get bad news again?

Monday, 24 October 2016 (day 0)

Surgery day. I got up at 5:15am. Arrived at the hospital at 7am, but surgery was scheduled for 1pm. Change of plan: my urology consultant said that on reviewing my MRI and histology report he thought it would be satisfactory to do a nerve-sparing procedure without lymph nodes dissection. Sounded like good news: the risk of complications should be a bit lower and recovery hopefully a bit faster. Let us hope the excision margins will be clear. I was a bit nervous. I also thought I

3

had easy veins, but the anaesthetist had to try twice. It was really nice to see both the urology consultant and the anaesthetist before the procedure, and to hear reassuring words from both of them.

I woke up at about 5pm in the recovery room and I had pain and nausea. I was transferred to the urology ward two hours later. Margherita, my wife, was there waiting for me. Unable to eat, I had sips of water through the night.

Tuesday, 25 October 2016 (day 1 post-op)

Intermittent sleep during the night. My abdomen was bloated and tender when I moved. Electric beds are great: I raised the back support when I wanted to sip water, then I lowered it again. I could not figure out how to stand up and walk. For breakfast I only managed a few spoonfuls of yogurt.

The nurse came to see me later in the morning and fitted a leg catheter bag; she then showed me how to drain it and how to connect to a larger night bag. She also encouraged me to stand up and sit on a chair, but I felt terribly sick and nauseous: I asked for some anti-nausea medication (I think they gave me some cyclizine) and returned to bed.

However, you need to be able to stand and walk, if you want to be discharged home, so I tried again on my own, just standing briefly and then a few steps. Each time a few more steps (to the window first, then to the door). I was in a urology ward, but none of the other five male patients in my bay seemed to be prostatectomy patients, probably because prostatectomy patients are discharged quickly.

It was now clear I had three challenges. Firstly, getting out of bed was difficult and painful. I had six abdominal wounds at the site where the robotic arms had been introduced. The normal way of getting out of bed using the abdominal muscles did not work: it caused real pain and it could cause surgical hernias. It seemed that the only way was turning on a side and then rising sideways. Even better if somebody helped me and pulled my arm. See pictures on how to get out of bed

4

at this website: https://healthonline.washington.edu/document/health_online/pdf/Activities-Daily-Living-After-Abdominal-Surgery.pdf

Secondly, I was really bloated with air in the abdominal cavity and inside the bowel. The bowel does not like surgery, it stops working and it fills with gas. To get better I needed to start passing wind and resolve the constipation. Easier said than done, as there is no specific effective medication. Rising from bed to sit and stand seemed to help and I tried to pass wind whenever I could (with modest results): I occasionally burped. Peppermint tea was recommended, but was not available in the ward. I tried to eat a bit for lunch but I only managed a soup and a few spoonfuls of fruit jelly.

The third problem was that when I stood or sat I had a really severe pain in the left shoulder (later in the right shoulder as well). Initially I thought I had pulled some muscles in my effort to rise from the bed sideways, but the nurse said it was due to my surgical procedure. I checked back the written explanatory note given to me weeks earlier: air is used to inflate the abdomen and allow the surgeons to operate and the residual trapped air can move just below the diaphragm and can cause referred pain to the shoulders! It really limited the time I could sit or stand, as the pain was severe. The pain disappeared if I laid back in bed, as the air presumably moved away from the diaphragm.

My urology consultant came to see me at lunchtime, I was really grateful for the visit and the update. He said that surgery was successful, though challenging, as there were adhesions between the prostate and the adjacent structures, due to the bleeding that took place after the transperineal prostatic biopsies. He confirmed that he spared both nerve bundles and the lymph nodes. The prognosis was good (I hoped he had not said this just to boost my morale), but we will know for sure only when the histology report becomes available. What I need (for the best probability of cure) is a report saying the tumour is entirely within the prostate with clear resection margins and no invasion of the seminal vesicles. The consultant also said I could go home later that day, no reason to stay for a second night, but I asked to stay because the pain was still severe when sitting or standing.

Wednesday, 26 October 2016 (day 2 post-op)

My wife Margherita drove me home in the late morning: this was a 40 minute journey. The difficult bit was getting in and out of the car, because of the abdominal pain, especially when I moved. When I got home I found a few "get better cards": one from some neighbours really captured the way I am (see below).

A list for Giuseppe:

1.	Get better soon
2.	Rest
3.	Get better soon
4.	Relax
5.	Get better soon
6.	Enjoy being looked after
7.	Get better soon
8.	Take it easy
9.	Get better soon
10.	Do what you are told
11.	Get better soon

I know how much you like lists!
Lots of love

I always like to plan, to consider all options in detail, and to make checklists. This strategy really applies well to all life scenarios, whether it is about buying a fridge or choosing a surgeon.

I sneezed once, it was very painful: I really hoped I would not get a respiratory or gastrointestinal infection over the next few weeks. I was terrified at the thought of having to cough or vomit. Still I had not had bowel movements since Monday despite the sodium docusate and the senna tablets from the hospital. The codeine given for pain control did not help in this respect, as it can cause constipation: I decided to manage the pain just with paracetamol (I thought I could, and the only strategy to control the shoulder pain was to lie down) and I decided to take some Movicol sachets as well (they had done a good job when I had been constipated after the prostatic biopsies).

Thursday, 27 October 2016 (day 3 post-op)

First bowel movement! It took three tablets of docusate sodium, three tablet of senna and three sachets of Movicol. This was good for the body and the spirit. The abdomen was still tender, but possibly a bit less bloated. Shoulder pains attributed to intraabdominal air were still a problem, when sitting and standing, but pain was less severe than two days earlier.

A friend came in to say hallo in the afternoon. It has always been so good to speak to him: he also had prostate cancer surgery a few years before, from which he had made a good recovery. As much as I find it useful to read books written by prostate cancer survivors, having a chat is so much better. And you can compare notes on how long it might take to recover and what is the best coping strategy. He told me he had felt much better, in a way, when he was able to tell all his friends and colleagues about his diagnosis and the treatment plan, so that they could understand why he had not been his usual self. Knowing there is a treatment plan always helps, and it helps when the date for surgery is set. Although there is usually no great urgency for the surgical procedure to be done immediately (the cancer usually evolves and progresses over months and years), if one has to have cancer surgery, one might as well do it soon, because then you know you have turned a corner and, although you will be initially unwell for a while after surgery, then the recovery begins, and surgery might be a cure.

I had a similar but not precisely identical experience. I also found it useful to tell friends and colleagues at an early stage. In fact, I told some of them even before the diagnosis was confirmed: a little bit of sympathy is always helpful, and talking to others is almost always good, it helps to clear your mind about what you want to do and you often get good tips and suggestions. The first five to seven days after my diagnosis was confirmed I was utterly demoralised and depressed, I cried a bit with my wife, I felt I was "drowning". I thought at some stage I should seek medical treatment for depression. Part of the problem was my "Italian" mentality: Italian patients often get all the radiology and histology reports immediately, even before seeing their specialist, thus (if they want) they can go to their specialist armed with information and a list of questions. I had gone to my specialist appointment, when a "robotic prostatectomy" was proposed, believing I still had a 50% chance of not even having cancer. And then, once given the diagnosis I was really worried: I was not worried primarily about the prostate cancer, which had not given me any trouble yet. I was really worried about the treatment options, all associated with unavoidable side-effects and consequences. And I felt I was a "prisoner of the system", and that things were happening to me regardless of my opinions and values. I had never wanted a PSA tests but I had been "tricked" into accepting one (it probably was a good thing I did it, but this is not how it felt at the time). I tried hard to avoid prostate biopsies and I pleaded for an MRI first: surely it would show nothing and I could ask for just further repeat PSA tests. Eventually, when the MRI showed a lesion in my prostate I had no other reasonable option but to accept the proposed prostatic biopsies. And then, with a confirmed prostate cancer diagnosis, I was told that on the basis of my age (60), history of ulcerative colitis (radiotherapy might be less well tolerated) and my Gleason score (3+4) and stage (probably stage two) I really should accept the offer of surgical treatment (robotic prostatectomy) rather than any of the radiotherapy options or androgen-deprivation therapy. In those difficult five to seven days of depression and despair, there were three things that kept me afloat: having a wonderful partner (my wife Margherita), being able to share my worries and concerns with friends and colleagues (many of them gave me useful tips) and going to the gym. I always felt I was at least a bit better after sweating in the gym and I had to be fit, if I was facing a major surgical procedure.

Part of my recovery from the depression process was to ask for a copy of all my relevant reports: MRI, bone scan and histology report. I got them five days after the outpatient appointment during which I had been told I had prostate cancer. Getting a copy of those reports made a lot of difference: I felt power and control were shifting towards me again. Armed with those reports I could do online searches for relevant publications, or just look up the treatment recommendations for patients with my cancer stage and grade in various textbooks. I also could seek a second opinion now that I had the reports. I decided to go and see a different urology surgeon: this was easy for me as I could ask a colleague working in my hospital. And so I did, I asked one of my colleagues who was recommended to me for his interpersonal skills: he was wonderful, he talked to me and my wife for 30 minutes and, armed with all the facts, I could now ask more relevant questions. I was particularly anxious to explore what might happen after surgery: surgery cannot guarantee a cure, adjuvant or salvage radiotherapy or androgen-deprivation therapy may still be required at a later stage. I felt I had preferred surgery over radiotherapy, but is it worthwhile choosing surgery over radiotherapy when there may be a risk of still needing radiotherapy after surgery? In that scenario, I would end up suffering from the cumulative consequences and side-effects of two types of treatment, not just one. I felt this was the most important choice I had ever had to make about my health during my life until that point: this was likely to affect the length and quality of my remaining life as well as my ability to fulfil my life goals. Although the second specialist visit had doubled my opportunities for asking questions, I thought I might as well seek a third and fourth opinion from specialists in a different country: sometimes there may be significant differences in approach and it might be interesting to hear about them. Between my bone scan and my biopsies I had spent a short holiday in Italy: I took the opportunity to go and see an eminent local specialist who also happened to be the chair of a European specialist body. It was an opportunity to go and see him for a chat, but I did not have at that time my reports: as agreed, I e-mailed my reports to him and he sent his treatment recommendation. I also phoned a friend who is a urologist based in Rome: we had a long telephone conversation. I also had chats with two friends who had undergone a radical prostatectomy (though not a robotic one) recently: they told me about their experiences. The second, third and fourth specialist recommended precisely what my urology consultant had recommended: a prostatectomy. My reading of the literature also suggested that surgery was probably the best option for me, or at least the option I disliked the least. Talking to the two friends who had undergone a prostatectomy was also extremely useful: they had recovered well and there were still prospects for a good life after prostatectomy, a life in which you can still have reasonable continence, do the things you like, even having a sex life. Now my morale changed and, while still a bit anxious about surgery, I was no longer depressed. The prostatectomy was no longer a procedure "imposed" on me: it was my choice, it was what I felt was the best option for me.

My only remaining reservations were about the precise surgical modalities. My surgeon had recommended removing at least one of the nerve bundles and had suggested that lymph node dissection should be considered. I was particularly worried about the lymph node dissection: it may carry some small additional risks and there may be no benefits in patients at low risk of lymph node involvement, but there could be significant benefits in high risk patients. I was thought to be an "intermediate" risk patient. Although the risk of significant side-effects from the lymph node dissection was low, there was a small risk. And maybe lymph node dissection would delay my surgical recovery, just at the time when an uneventful timely recovery would be so good at boosting moral. So, should I let my surgeon know that I had concerns or preferences about the possible lymph node dissection? After extensive searches and reading I had some level of knowledge on this but, as we all know, sometimes having a little knowledge can be a dangerous thing. It would have been presumptuous of me to think that I knew better than a very experienced urology consultant.

In the end, what I did was to write a one-page letter to my consultant. I was not telling him what to do, I had trust in his judgment, I was telling him about my fears and my values. This is what I said in my letter about the proposed lymph node dissection:

> I have concerns regarding the proposed lymph node dissection, being aware of the possible unpleasant, though infrequent, complications. I am particularly worried about obturator nerve or vascular injury, and a little bit about lymphocele. I did a bit of reading about this: I understand that there is some uncertainty about the benefit especially in American studies, but some other studies suggest there is a benefit. If there is a benefit, it seems to be more significant

in the high-risk cases, but might also apply to intermediate-risk cases (like me). On this, again, I trust your judgement and would accept the lymph node dissection if you think it is in my best interest. Can I just express a preference for not taking the lymph node dissection to extremes, especially if you felt there was a risk of morbidity in any particular circumstances during the procedure?

Thank you for accepting me as a patient. I realise that, as a healthcare worker, I may be a more difficult patient. I must admit that this diagnosis has really demoralised me, but I hope to turn the corner and I find it helpful if I can be kept informed and have the opportunity to voice any concerns.

In some way I was relieved when, on the day of surgery, my urology consultant said that on reviewing my MRI and histology report he felt in my case the risk of extension to the lymph nodes was less than 5%, hence the lymph node excision was not necessary.

Friday, 28 October 2016 (day 4 post-op)

I have checked my weight today: 86 kg, down from about 89 kg before surgery. Well, I am a tall man, thus for me 89 kg is equivalent to a Body Mass Index of 25 (within the recommended 20–25 optimal range). I had not eaten at all on Monday and very little on Tuesday. In the previous two days I managed small snacks but not full meals, as I felt bloated. I had tried to compensate the small content of each meal with having more meal times, and eating seemed to be a way of reducing the abdominal bloating. I am just about resuming my normal eating habits.

First shower!

Sunday, 30 October 2016 (day 6 post-op)

First brief walk out of the house to post a letter. Giacomo, my younger son came with me: he had come back from Cambridge (where he works) to spend the weekend with his dad (and mum). Is this an opportunity to find out what his life plans are?

Monday, 31 October 2016 (day 7 post-op)

The catheter was removed in the morning and I passed the subsequent TWOC (Trial Without Catheter) test: an ultrasound scan taken just after I had been to the loo showed minimal residual urine volume in the bladder, meaning I could empty the bladder well and there was no risk of urinary retention.

Now the battle for continence begins! I was given pads to wear inside the pants. It does not seem to be the worst possible incontinence scenario: the urethra is not quite an open tap. I have multiple urine leaks either on moving or coughing or when I first feel a stimulus, but they are small volume leaks.

I was given a prescription for Sildenafil (Viagra) 50mg on alternate days to continue for six months: this is part of the penile rehabilitation plan.

Ah, the pleasure of a long shower without a dangling catheter and a urinary bag strapped to the leg!

Tuesday, 1 November 2016 (day 8 post-op)

It is great to wear ordinary trousers again, and not the loose tracksuit bottoms I was wearing all the time before, in order to accommodate the catheter and the urine bag strapped to the leg.

But now I have to wear continence pads to cope with the post-prostatectomy urinary incontinence. There seems to be a clear pattern. Just a few small leaks in the morning, but more frequent episodes in the afternoon and evening. I am still on the search for the optimal most suitable type of pad.

Wednesday, 2 November 2016 (day 9 post-op)

I woke up a few times during the night with painful bladder cramps; the haemauria (red colour of the urine due to the presence of blood) is ongoing, though intermittent and minimal.

I went for a walk and came back with slightly wet trousers: the issue is the targeted positioning of the continence pads. The penis is in the habit of "roaming" and falling downside beyond the edge of the Tena For Men level 2 pad, but larger pads are uncomfortable and I do not need the capacity to absorb large volumes of urine. I phoned the prostate cancer UK survivorship nurse: amongst other things she gives advice on regaining the ability to have sexual intimacy. She will give me an appointment for some time in December or January.

I feel that I need to plan what I want to do in the near future and for the rest of my life. Is the prostate cancer an alarm bell alerting me to the need to review my plans and aspirations? First of all, I need to have a clear idea about what my objectives are. The list of short-intermediate term goals I have put together is as shown in Table 1.

Table 1. Reflection on my short and intermediate term life objectives.	
Objective	How to achieve it
Achieving better control of the urine incontinence	• Pelvic floor exercises • Study the choice of different continence pads and how best to position them • Will get better with time
Regaining the ability to have sexual intimacy	• Just started "penile rehabilitation" with sildenafil • Specialist nurse appointment in January • Will get better with time • Intimacy is not just about penetration
Regaining physical fitness	• Going for walks (the only physical activity I am currently allowed) • Continue with healthy diet • Resume gym work and classes in full eight weeks after my prostatectomy, but lighter careful work can start earlier
Establishing whether I will need radiotherapy or androgen-deprivation therapy after the prostatectomy	• My first outpatient appointment will be about eight weeks after surgery: histology will be the key result and then the follow-up PSA tests • I can quantify the relapse risk now by using the appropriate online nomogram

(continued)

13

Table 1. Reflection on my short and intermediate term life objectives – *continued.*	
Objective	How to achieve it
I have now realised anything can happen at any time in my life: I need to make the best of life and enjoy every day ("carpe diem", Horace 23BC)	• Plan holiday with Margherita, possibly in February–March (I had to cancel the summer holiday because of the biopsies: I am "due" a holiday) • Plan week-end trips to London and Cambridge to make sure we keep in touch with our sons who live there • Find a way to spend more time with friends • Make new friends • Look again at the list of things I would like to do whilst I am still an energetic man (the list currently includes: writing a book, digitalising the family collections of pictures, finding out if I am really hopeless at dancing, some far-away holidays, serious gardening, cookery classes to expand my repertoire in the kitchen)
Look again at the retirement plan: I am 60, my original plan was to retire at the age of 65, but I could retire now if I accept a lower pension	• Attend Retirement Seminar in December • Meet with Independent Financial Advisor in January • I need to know first what is the likely course of my prostate cancer: am I cured? Am I likely to see a relapse? • If I retire now I might miss the social interactions I have at work: thus, consider the intermediate option of retiring and going back to work part-time

Friday, 4 November (day 11 post-op)

In the past few nights I woke two or three times with cramp-like pains relieved by emptying the bladder. It was not like that before the prostatectomy. The written instructions I was given for the prostatectomy refer to "bladder spasms" occurring while you have a catheter. Well, I only suffered from this after the catheter was removed.

I have noticed this entry at healing.well.com from a patient who had a prostatectomy four months earlier: "With a full bladder I develop lots of pain until I relieve myself. The act of urination does not hurt; in fact the stream flow is quite good. However, the pain when the bladder is full causes a kind of intense stinging pain in the bladder area. When this happens, it is very painful just to walk to bathroom. I still have minor stress incontinence". This is precisely my situation, though much earlier after surgery: during the day I empty my bladder frequently, during the nights it fills up and does not like it! I hope it will resolve with time.

Saturday, 5 November (day 12 post-op)

Agostino, my older son, came from London to spend the weekend with us. We are planning to go for an afternoon tea in town later on.

I still have painful spasms both during the day and the night, after I have emptied my bladder. Is this a urinary tract infection (UTI) or a consequence of surgery? I did not have this problem the first few days after the catheter removal. I decide to go to an urgent care centre: I have a positive dipstick test (red cell, leukocytes, protein were detected), which is consistent with but not absolute proof of a UTI. The abnormal dipstick results could just be due to the recent surgery. The urine has been sent for urine culture (two to three days for the result) and I have been started on an antibiotic (trimethoprim). About 75% of the UTIs in the UK respond to trimethoprim. This is a disruption on my road to recovery, but you know what they say: the road to recovery is often a bumpy road.

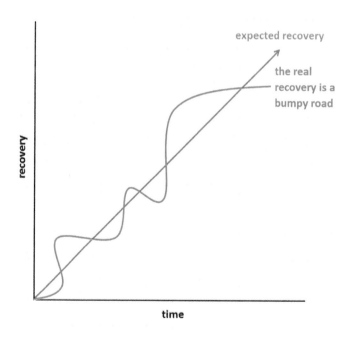

Figure 1. The road to recovery is a bumpy road.

Monday, 6 November (day 13 post-op)

No response to trimethoprim: during the night I got up every hour to pee, some nine to 10 times in total. And every time it is agony. The pain, or spasm, is stronger just after I finish weeing. In between episodes of peeing I have just minimal discomfort.

The plan is:

a) Could be a UTI but some 30% of bacteria causing UTIs are resistant to trimethoprim. I need to book appointment with my family doctor.
b) I need to speak to the nurse who checked my urine residual volume in the bladder last week; maybe we need to check again I do not have urinary retention.
c) I feel I need to start exercising again, but I was told to take it easy for the first six weeks. To go up and down the stairs and start using the exercise tube.

Wednesday, 9 November (day 16 post-op)

Somewhat demoralised today. I have frequency and I go to the toilet every hour during the day or two hours during the night, but the real problem is the painful micturition: I have a very intense pain that starts at the end of the micturition and continues for about a minute after. The urine sample showed leukocytes in the urine (pyuria) but no bacteria were cultured. Antibiotics: I had trimethoprim first, then co-amoxiclav. Neither has made any difference. Urine alkalinisation with Cystopurin has made no difference either. I have gone back to the urology clinic to check the post-void bladder volume: no evidence at all of retention.

Not sure what to do next, other than going back to my family doctor and ask for a urology referral (if the problem persists).

Thursday, 10 November (day 17 post-op)

Back to the gym for the first time: very light session.

Urethral pain after micturition continues. The pain started after I started penile rehabilitation with phosphodiesterase type 5 inhibitors.

Yesterday I was getting better but it got worse after the bedtime dose. Was it because the penile tumescence was stretching the urethral sutures? It could be just coincidence, but I think I will stop the penile rehabilitation medications for one week.

Saturday, 12 November (day 19 post-op)

Three of my friends have come over from Italy to see me, they will stay until Monday. Two ladies and a man. We used to go out together when most of us were at university in Bologna, we were part of a group of 10–15 friends. Is the old gang back in action? I cannot go with them on long walks (I am getting tired easily) but tomorrow we will all go to Seaham Hall for a traditional English high tea.

Tuesday, 15 November (day 22 post-op)

Back to the gym for the second time since surgery: I have not felt like wanting to exercise in the past days. I could not quite put my finger on it, but I did not feel completely well: I had a mild sore throat (viral infection?), rectal discomfort where the prostate was, especially if I sat or stood for long (I have tried cold packs, is there a haematoma deep down there?), not feeling very energetic and if I went out I could easily feel quite cold (I needed a really hot shower to recover). But in the morning, especially if the sun is out, I feel at my best, this is the time for gentle exercise.

Continence-wise, things are better. The first few days after the catheter was removed I mainly had stress incontinence with multiple small leaks when bending, coughing or getting tired later in the day. Then for a period of days I also had urge incontinence: I tried not think about emptying my bladder until when I was right in front of the toilet and ready to go, or else I lost control. But now I am better, especially during the night. Last night I had a six-hour break without going to the toilet. The pain after emptying my bladder (bladder spasm or urethral burning?) is still there during the day (strangely not during the night) but seems less intense.

Sunday, 20 November (day 27 post-op)

I have completed today the 28th, and last, tinzaparin (anticoagulant) injection. Hooray! A friend of mine though, who had an open prostatectomy, had a deep vein thrombosis some two months after surgery and it really set him back. Maybe I will continue with the anti-embolic leg stockings for a bit longer. Also, I am back into exercises. I have been to the gym on seven of the past eight days, but I only do light work: in particular, I am trying not to do anything that stresses the abdomen. I prefer the gym to going for a walk: in the gym you can see people and have a chat, and the toilet is nearby if you need it. Maybe my wounds are still healing, and I do not want a surgical site hernia, thus I am careful not to do anything to cause pain or stretch the abdominal muscles. On the treadmill I walk, uphill as well, but I have not started running yet.

Tuesday, 22 November (day 29 post-op)

I went to the first meeting of the Prostate Cancer Support Group, which gave me an opportunity to ask questions about continence. There were more men with a history of radiotherapy and/or androgen deprivation therapy than prostatectomy: I guess most prostatectomy men think they have sorted it out, and want to forget about their prostate cancer. Conversely, I hope for the best but I like to plan for the worst. If I will ever need androgen-deprivation therapy, I want to know about it and how to mitigate the side-effects. My experience of the National Health Service (NHS) in the UK is that you cannot exert choices or express preferences unless you put an effort into informing yourself well before that information is needed.

NHS appointments are like really important executive meetings to which you are invited, sometimes to make important decisions about your health, but you are not sent an agenda or any relevant information prior to the meeting. Then, when you are there, you are told that you have prostate cancer or that after your prostatectomy your PSA has gone up. And then they will say: we want to refer you for this or for that treatment. It is difficult to give informed consent in these circumstances: if I had known the results beforehand I would have prepared,

I would have searched the internet, I would have made a list of appropriate questions, I could express preferences. I suppose you could say you want to think and discuss it again at a subsequent appointment (if they offer you one), but there are limited opportunities for this in the NHS.

Or else, you must arm yourself with as much information as possible about every conceivable scenario before your next outpatient appointment. Still I think that, if the outpatient appointment was like a company executive board meeting, everybody would agree this is a dysfunctional way to operate and you could not expect meaningful important decisions to be taken in this way. The initial cancer diagnosis may have to be given face-to-face, but for subsequent appointments, how about getting the agenda first, perhaps in the form a letter saying: *these are your prostatectomy histology results, in your circumstances we would consider radiotherapy and we will discuss this at your next appointment.*

Wednesday, 23 November (day 30 post-op)

Last night was the first night I have not needed to get up and empty my bladder. Daytime continence also seems to be a bit better.

I have received a letter today from my urology consultant regarding my prostatectomy histology report: the report is not as good as I hoped it would be. The final Gleason grade is slightly higher: 4+3, not 3+4 as in the biopsy histology, this is a bit worse. More importantly, the cancer extended outside the prostate capsule and reached the resection margin. I suspect I am heading for salvage radiotherapy but it all depends on whether and when the PSA goes up; I believe my first check will be on 20 December. How extensive was the contact with the resection margin? This can affect the prognosis. Was there inflammation as well as cancer? I would like to see my full histology report: this is what defines my prognosis now. I have just written to my consultant asking for a copy of the full report: it sounds as if there will be critical decisions to make and I want to be fully informed. Also, I would need this report, if I ever wanted a second opinion.

Friday, 2 December (day 39 post-op)

I went to a retirement seminar. I am considering retiring in the second half of next year (2017). I am not sure though whether just to retire, or retire and go back to work part-time. The latter seems to be the best of both worlds, provided I remain in good health and do not have to struggle with the side-effects of a possible future radiotherapy.

Saturday, 3 December (day 40 post-op)

I went to the gym Christmas party for a couple of hours. I was very undecided about whether go or not. Seeing friends, and having a laugh, would be good. But friends ask questions: how did the surgery go? And what would I say? It had not gone as well as I hoped and I seem to be at high risk of a relapse. No immediate threat to my life, but a greater probability of more unpleasant treatment including perhaps, eventually, the dreaded androgen deprivation. The bottom line is: sympathy is great but I do not want pity.

I got the impression some men with prostate cancer retreat into social isolation, or just do not want to discuss prostate cancer at all with others.

Monday, 5 December (day 42 post-op)

First day back at work! The plan is to work just in the morning for the first week, then a bit of lunchtime exercise and I will drive back home whilst it is still daylight.

I have now received a copy of my prostatectomy histology report: the key additional piece of information is that the estimated extent of the positive resection margin (the length in which the cancer cells reach, and possibly extend beyond, the edge of the removed tissue) was 10 mm anteriorly. On a quick review of the literature, it seems that the risk of relapse is higher when the positive resection margin is more than 3 mm as in my case; conversely having positive margins on the anterior surface of the prostate may carry a slightly reduced risk.

Wednesday, 21 December (day 58 post-op)

So, yesterday I had my first post-op check, and I phoned today to find out what the PSA result was: undetectable! They use a sensitive (but not the most sensitive) test: undetectable means less than 0.02 ng/ml. However, because of the extracapsular extension and positive surgical margins, the long-term probability of relapse (biochemical relapse) is 79% within 10 years: I did the relapse risk calculation using the Memorial Sloan Kettering Cancer Center post-radical prostatectomy nomogram. The longer the PSA remains undetectable, the better my chances will become. Next PSA test will be in April, six months post-surgery.

So, what are my treatment goals now?

- My primary aspiration is to be in that 21% group of patients who, despite having the same prostate cancer features as me, do not relapse. I can probably improve my odds a little bit with exercise, diet, Pomi-T, aspirin and a bit of fighting spirit.
- If I failed the primary goal, I hope at least not to relapse in the first two years after surgery: according to my nomogram, my chances of achieving this currently are 59%. I need to work on maximising my chances to achieve at least the secondary goal.
- Thirdly, I need to work on physical fitness, so that I am ready to face the next challenge (radiotherapy) if it will be necessary.
- Fourthly, if I relapsed even after radiotherapy, I would need androgen deprivation therapy: I would need to put together a strategy to minimise the side effects of this. In essence, it is always a good strategy to have contingency plans. I think good generals always have a plan B (and plans C, D, E as well) whilst working with determination on winning with plan A.

Physically I am fine, though in the gym I still take it easy with any exercises involving the abdominal muscles: sometimes it is still slightly painful around the wounds, and I guess it is better to regain fitness gradually, whilst minimising the risk of surgical site hernias. Urinary continence is variable, recently I had a cold: it was a disaster as I "leaked" with every sneeze or cough. Am I getting more continent? To try to answer this question I have started weighing the continence pads (weight when removed minus original dry weight) to estimate the amount of urine leaked over 24-hours (this is known as a 24-hour pad test): the amount is pretty variable on a daily basis and a weekly average might be more meaningful. I hope to see an improvement over the next few months. Yesterday I was also told it would be fine to try to resume sexual activity.

Friday, 13 January (day 81 post-op)

Physically, I am almost back to my pre-surgical level of fitness. I have re-joined all the gym classes I used to go to. Urinary continence is improving, as proven by the 24-hour pad test: in mid-December I was leaking over 80 grams of urine per day, in part because of a nasty cold as I had stress incontinence with every sneeze or cough. Over the subsequent two weeks the amount of urine leaked into the pads went down to just over 40 grams per day, and in the past week it was on average 20 grams per day. The aim of complete (or almost complete) urinary continence recovery seems realistic.

As far as erectile function is concerned, it is work in progress. Sexual intercourse is more difficult, though possible: but I think that, as for the urinary incontinence, there is scope for further improvement over the next months. I will discuss all aspects of recovery at my appointment with the prostate cancer survivorship specialist nurse. I hope I can achieve my goals with grit, determination and willingness to explore a range of strategies.

The story of my life

Il Resto del Carlino is the local regional newspaper of Bologna, the Italian city where I was born and where I attended the medical school. In Italy, it used to be like that: if you were born in a University town, that is where you studied. I have a paper cutting from *Il Resto del Carlino* dated 13 November 1979: it says that the day before the oral exams for Surgery (of the Bologna University medical school) were taking place. That is the way it was: oral exams, a test of memory (I would say regurgitation from textbooks) and theoretical knowledge, not of clinical skills. It was common practice that, after the oral examination, the examiners would offer you a mark: if you felt the mark did not reflect your knowledge and would affect your average score (the final graduation mark would take into account the average of all the many oral exams) you could turn the mark down and reattend the next examination session usually one month later. It had always been done like that in all the exams: it was the only way to fight back against an educational system that valued retaining bits of information over critical thinking or clinical skills. The medical course in Italy was six years, as opposed to five in the UK, but if you chose so you could get through with seeing very few patients and just studying from books. I was completely disillusioned, not only did I dislike the complete lack of practical clinical content and practice, but also I disliked a good numbers of the academic doctors in the university hospital. They were not like most other doctors in non-teaching hospital or general practice: a significant proportion of them had a complete lack of respect for the students and, not infrequently, lack of respect and good manners with patients. Those bad teachers had achieved academic power in the most prestigious hospital in the region: only two things usually mattered to them, publications to increase their academic prestige, and private practice. Teaching students was a nuisance, the less the better, and patients were just fodder.

The paper cutting of the newspaper dated 13 November said that at the beginning of the Surgery oral examination the Professor had asked all the students to sign the examination records: that meant that whatever mark he would offer, it would be recorded without the option of declining and re-attending another examination session. That was not the way we had done any other exams: the students refused to sign and the Professor refused to start the oral exams. At that stage, says the paper cutting, a medical student sat on the desk behind which the examiners were and then all the other students followed suit and there was a general sit-in, which prevented the exams from taking pace. Later on, says the newspaper, a delegation of 70 students went to meet the university vice-chancellor who explained that the professor of surgery had followed the university procedures to the letter, though those procedures had not been enacted since 1968 (1968 is when the first rebellious wave amongst students had started).

The oral exams for Surgery restarted one week later, and the students were not asked to sign the examination records before a mark had been offered. That student protest must be seen in the context of Italy (and France I believe): since the late 1960s into well into the 1990s it was common for students to have political ideas, to protest and dispute, sit-ins were common both in secondary schools and universities. The student, who had started this particular protest, by sitting on the professor desk, was me. When my father found out, he told me I was finished and that I would never graduate. He was too pessimistic, I still graduated and with full marks. But I had already made up my mind: the Italian system was not for me. I knew very well how it worked (we all knew, but most accepted it), advancement was not through merit but through patronage of a few influential professors or heads of department in non-teaching hospitals (they were known as "barons"), or political patronage. Corruption in the healthcare system was not uncommon, inefficiency was the rule. I was a rebel, I would never fit in. I decided that after my graduation I would do my year in the army and then I would leave and work abroad.

Early in 1983 I was a trainee in Orthopaedics, as was common at the time I was unpaid (trainees were not paid in the first few years) and not being trained much either. I was really just biding my time, waiting for the compulsory service in the army to start, then I would leave. I met Margherita in a club in Bologna, I think it was the evening of 23 January 1983. Not that I liked disco dancing, I just went for socialising. Margherita was quite a beautiful girl and independent-minded. Actually, I had met her just once before in a clothing shop, she was there with some mutual male friends and was buying some leopard print thing. I had heard about her via these mutual friends, all studying electronic engineering: Margherita was just one of a small number of female students on that course. I was under the impression that she had a boyfriend. In the club she was with a male friend but not a boy-friend. In my experience opportunities often do not present a second time in life. I decided to go over and chat her up, but I needed a chat up line. So, I went over and asked if she would come to live with me in the UK, we started dating the day after.

We left Italy for good on 2 January 1985: I had finished my service in the army in September 1984, Margherita graduated later in 1984. We left with my small Fiat 127 car and drove all the way to Calais. We arrived there in the evening and there was a storm. We had booked our Channel crossing with a hovercraft and there it was, it came in the dark (lights on) through the storm floating over the sea and then over the land. It was quite an experience. During the crossing I was sick because of the rough sea. The day after we drove to Southampton: I had a contact there with a promise of an unpaid attachment to get experience and familiarise myself with the British healthcare system. All my friends were confident we would be back in Italy within a few months: I never went back (except for holidays). My first regular job started in August 1985 as a Senior House Officer in Pathology (in Italy my graduation thesis had been in histopathology). I then proposed to Margherita, and we got married in 1986.

Our two sons were born in London: Agostino in 1991, Giacomo in 1993. Agostino was born at St Mary's Hospital where I was working as a Senior Registrar in Medical Microbiology. A few months after Agostino had been born, I became unwell: malaise, headache, inter-mittent sore throat and fever. Sounded like a viral respiratory infection but it went on, and on. After two weeks I sought the opinion of a consultant in infectious diseases, various tests were arranged and eventually I was briefly admitted to hospital, 24 days after the onset, for the investigation of what was regarded as a pyrexia of unknown origin. When no cause is found one starts getting worried, as there is the possibility of either a severe infection, like tuberculosis, or a malignant tumour as the cause of the prolonged febrile illness. At last the cause was found: it was a virus called Cytomegalovirus! I had it in my blood and my son had it in his urine. Serology showed my wife had evidence of having acquired the infection earlier in her life but not recently. Thus, we could piece together the likely sequence of events. Cytomegalovirus is a common infection, similar to infectious mononucleosis, and it can cause rather protracted symptoms (five weeks in my case). My wife had had the infection earlier in her life: pregnant women can reactivate the infection and can pass on the virus to the baby, but in the context of reactivation they also pass on protective antibodies, hence the babies are often asymptomatic but excrete the virus in their urine. Fathers, if they have not suffered from the infection before, can get the infection from their infant children, possibly when changing the nappies. It had been unpleasant but all was good in the end. But after the pain, could I get some gain from this experience? I decided to write up this story as a case report in a medical journal, to share the learning points, and so it was the article was published.[1]

On the whole, my health has been good. In 1997 I was diagnosed with ulcerative colitis but it has been easily controlled with mesalazine, a well-tolerated medication. In 2016 I turned 60, my wife, who is one year younger, decided to retire that year. My plan was to carry on working full time for another five years. But then, unexpectedly, I was diagnosed with prostate cancer. This has been the greatest health challenge in my life so far. And now I am rethinking my life plans. I have had surgery, but it is too soon to say whether I am cured for good or whether I have just passed the first hurdle. Do I need to change my life plan and make time for other things in my life, things other than work? And how do I maximise my chances of winning the battle with prostate cancer?

A rough guide for prostatectomy patients: how to deal with problems and get better outcomes

I am not a prostate cancer specialist, I am a patient, but I have reflected on my diagnosis and treatment, and whenever possible I have asked questions or searched for information from a variety of sources. If you want a comprehensive specialist book on prostate cancer, look elsewhere. There are books written by specialists specifically to educate or guide patients: the one written by Dr Chodak is an excellent one.[2] There are also books written for a medical audience, including a recent comprehensive textbook[3] and there are many relevant articles in medical journals: many patients are able to make sense of the key messages in these sources, particularly if they make an effort to conquer the terminology.

What you will find in this part of my book is different: this is my own take on what practical problems can be encountered and what might be important determinants of good outcomes. The emphasis is on what we can do for ourselves, how we can take charge and make informed choices and how we can maximise our chances of good outcomes. Whenever possible I have tried to be evidence-based and to provide references to back up some of the statements made in this section of the book, or else I will tell you that all I am offering is my own personal interpretation or opinion.

Throughout this book, I will also refer frequently to the experience of other prostate cancer patients who have chronicled their battle in published books.[4–8] There is a lot to be learnt from them.

I hope this book will be of interest to other prostate cancer patients. However, this book has also been written for the benefit of my two sons, or indeed any other close male relatives (brothers and sons) of prostate cancer patients. Brothers and sons are at increased risk, but can reduce the risk by changing their lifestyles and will probably want to undertake PSA screening. But, before you undertake PSA screening, you need to ponder first about the risks and benefits of screening and how screening fits with your outlook on life. Even more important is to be well-informed about how you want to manage your PSA results, and you really need to do this before your first PSA test. Do not fall into one of many traps: rash decisions, unjustified panic, uninformed choices, not making use of recent advances or new technologies, over-treatment or undertreatment. Get information now and be ahead of the curve!

I would also encourage you to use Google Scholar, whenever you have a particular topic or issue you want to explore: you can use Google Scholar to search for appropriate medical articles. There are various online sources of information on how to use Google Scholar, see for instance http://www.otago.ac.nz/library/pdf/Google_Scholar_Tips. pdf You need to think of appropriate key words and perhaps combine them with AND or OR. Let us say you want to find out articles about deep vein thrombosis after robotic prostatectomy, enter: *deep vein thrombosis AND robotic prostatectomy*. You will then get links to a list of articles: some the links will take you to the full text article (often in pdf format) without charge, with other links you may only get the abstract. If you are given only the abstract and you want the full text, there is usually a way to pay for access to the full article. Sometimes you need to visit the website of the medical journal that published the article, enter the article details and pay for the access. Your local librarian may be able to help. All hospitals have medical librarians who are very competent at retrieving medical articles, or at least at giving explanations.

Personally, I do my medical literature searches using Ovid Medline (better than Google Scholar) but access is via subscription: healthcare employers or healthcare associations give access to Ovid Medline (or similarly sophisticated search engines). Certain libraries may be able to give access.

Depression

Demoralisation and depression are common responses to a diagnosis of cancer and they can be exacerbated by a lack of family or social support. Dr Scholz, in his book co-written with prostate cancer patient Ralph Blum, warns about the possible dangers of biopsies: *biopsy itself is not particularly dangerous but the psychological impact of a cancer diagnosis is monumental.*[4] Sometimes depression can be a transient self-resolving problem (this was my personal experience), but serious or protracted depression needs medical treatment.

Daniel Carlson in his book, in which he recounts his prostate cancer story, reports his reaction to the diagnosis.[7] *My reaction to being told that I have prostate cancer ran along several predictable avenues... surprise... shock... fear... and a fear of being alone with this new reality in my life. But then, again, like many men, I quickly learned that there is a sizeable community of others who have dealt with this disease and, unbeknownst to me, this group included a number of my friends and acquaintances.*

David Thomas, another prostate cancer patient who has written about his story, suffered even more from depression, initially because of social isolation.[6] After the diagnosis *I had several sleepless nights... The trouble was, I didn't feel I could tell any of those close to me. I was separated from my wife... I did not feel I could tell my children... I didn't feel able to tell my mother or my sister. I didn't have any close friends.* Eventually David e-mailed a childhood friend, who he thought would be sympathetic, and she replied and that made him feel a bit better. David found a way of turning from depression into a fighting spirit mood, and then he told all his family members. David, though, had advanced prostate cancer and was put on androgen-deprivation medi-cations, which caused ongoing unpleasant side-effects: this can take a toll on even the strongest fighting spirit. *I'd had so many things go wrong – my marriage had broken up, my dad had died, and I was seriously ill. It all caught up with me... I just felt completely alone, and I got more and more miserable.* Eventually, on visiting his daughter, his wife, from whom he was separated, recognised the depression symptoms and took him to the family doctor, who prescribed antidepressants. But antidepressants can take some time to work. On one day he was feeling suicidal and called the Samaritans' helpline, and then his cat came back, while he was on the phone, and started miaowing: things started changing for the better.

UK residents may want to go on the *Clinical Depression – NHS choices* website: there is some guidance on recognising depression and when to see a family doctor. There is also a link to an online screening test (http://www.nhs.uk/Tools/Pages/depression.aspx) that tells you if you are likely to suffer from depression. In the USA a similar online test can be found at http://www.mentalhealthamerica.net/mental-health-screen/patient-health

There are similar depression websites for many countries in the local languages.

There is quite a body of medical literature on depression in men with prostate cancer. Patients with cancer, understandably, are more likely to develop either depression or anxiety. Depression can occur as a result of receiving a prostate cancer diagnosis, or later on in the prostate cancer journey: depression may be more common in those men undergoing androgen-deprivation therapy or at a more advanced stage of the disease, and might be less common in men with a partner. Marriage can be beneficial in reducing psychological distress bur only when there is high partner support.[9] O'Shaughnessy and others also found that wives or partners are a key psychosocial support to men with prostate cancer and may also provide a valuable insight into men's supportive care needs, which men are often unable to recognize themselves.[10] If you want to know if a man with prostate cancer is suffering from depression, you may be better off asking his partner, says Ralph Blum in his book, as women are providers of more accurate information about their man's emotional state: *We ask, 'Have you been feeling sad or depressed?' and he goes, 'No, not at all.' Then we ask the spouse, and she says, 'Yes, he's depressed all the time.'*[4]

Depression in men with prostate cancer may have significant deleterious consequences: Jayadevappa and others have shown that depression is associated with an increase in emergency room visits, hospitalisations, outpatient visits and mortality.[11] The reason for poorer outcomes in patients with depression has also been explored in an article by Prasad and others: they reported that men with depression are less likely to undergo definitive therapy such as surgery or radiation.[12]

So, it is important to recognise depression and treat it appropriately. The two main therapies are antidepressants and cognitive behavioural therapy (a talking therapy). However, there are other beneficial things that men with depression can do! Exercise, for example, is well recognised for its beneficial effect on depression. Spirituality, which is defined as helping one understand and find purpose and meaning in life, can exists both inside or outside any religious framework and it seems to reduce depression in prostate cancer patients.[13]

Rachel Carlyle in an article published in the Weekend Body + Soul insert of *The Times* (Saturday 26 November 2016) lists the seven activities that research suggest are most likely to make people happy. The list includes:

- Gardening.
- Eating more yoghurt and pickled vegetables (more healthy bacteria in your gut).
- Scottish dancing (or other line dancing).
- Giving to charity.
- Walking in the woods.
- Team sports.
- Getting a dog.

I am not surprised that gardening features in the list: it combines exercise, exposure to the sun, being a purposeful activity, and satisfaction from growing your own produce or having a nice plant display.

Choosing the treatment modality or the surgeon

A diagnosis of prostate cancer may bring about the need for making a number of decisions: which treatment modality, which treatment centre, which urology surgeon or which other specialist. Or maybe not, you could choose to ask your family doctor to recommend a treatment centre and specialist, and you may ask the specialist to recommend what he/she thinks is the best treatment modality. What you will do might depend on your personality, on the information you have and on the influence of other people around you. There may be problems with an entirely passive approach. If you go to different treatment centres, or different specialists, you may get different treatment modalities recommendations, and there may sometimes be significant differences in the proportion of satisfactory outcomes. And if you do not seek information about the possible consequences and complications of different treatment modalities, how can you explain to your specialist which of those consequences you would rather minimise, which may have a substantial influence on any treatment modality recommendation?

All specialists are to some extend biased. Dr Chodak in chapter 17 of his book reports this anecdote: years ago, a survey was done in which both urologists and radiation oncologists were asked what treatment they would recommend for a 60-year-old family member with localised prostate cancer: nearly all the surgeons recommended surgery and nearly all the radiation therapists recommended radiation.[2]

But is it really possible to exercise choice? The diagnostic process is not always geared towards giving you many opportunities for choice. And let us be frank: many health systems, and certainly the National Health Service in the UK, are under a lot of pressure. Giving patients the option of exercising choice means extending consultation times or arranging further consultations. In my case I had an outpatient appointment to discuss my prostate biopsy results: on the basis on my previous PSA results I thought I had only a 39% chance of having cancer. Then during the course of just one consultation I was told that I had cancer (shock), that the cancer grade was Gleason 7 (4+3 on one side, 3+4 on the other), that cancer had been found in 11 out of

42 biopsy cores with the overall core volume with tumour being 10%, that given my history of ulcerative colitis surgery would be preferable to radiotherapy, that consideration should be given to removing at least one nerve bundle (though it can worsen erectile function) and to do lymph node dissection (though it can increase the risk of side effects) and that surgery could be arranged on a proposed date four weeks later.

There was a lot to take in, including a blow to morale. I had tried to think prior to this appointment what questions I would ask in relation to each possible scenario: but there were too many scenarios to consider, such as no cancer but need to repeat the biopsies in future, or the scenario of a less aggressive cancer Gleason 6 for which possibly active surveillance might be acceptable, or even worse scenarios with Gleason scores equal or above 8. In the end, I tried to do the sensible think: I asked some questions, and so did my wife, I asked for a copy of all my reports (MRI, bone scan, biopsies histology) and I agreed to have surgery four weeks later: I thought the four weeks grace time would be enough for me to ponder over those reports, look up the literature and ask for a second and third opinion). If I decided to stick with surgery I was already confident I had chosen a good surgeon, thus I had no hesitations in that respect. For me it was extremely important to get a copy of my radiology and histology reports, which allowed me to seek appropriate information and further opinions: I felt I was in charge again. Xu also reported that some men diagnosed with prostate cancer *reported coping with the distress by attempting to take control of the decision making process.*[14]

Jay Cohen in his book describes an experience similar to mine: prostatic biopsies conducted because of his raised PSA had shown a Gleason 6 cancer, which is regarded as low grade and unlikely to metastasize, and he had been referred by his urologist to a prostate surgeon.[5] The prostate surgeon recommended a prostatectomy, with removal of one or both neurovascular bundles, and explained there was some risk of erectile dysfunction and incontinence but there could be "some return" of normal sexual and urinary function "over time". Mr Cohen initially felt too dumbfounded to answer the question as to whether he agreed to the surgical plan, but then mouthed a feeble yes. However, there was a three month waiting list for surgery, which gave him the opportunity to join some support groups: as the official hospital support group was not meeting that month, he ended up in an independent group of men, all cancer survivors, who regularly met to support each other, share information and discuss any new publications on prostate cancer. Mr Cohen then found out that it was debatable whether he should have a prostatectomy, that actives surveillance would be acceptable for a Gleason 6 case like him, if one is prepared to accept the risk that biopsies sometimes do not give the right grade, and he learnt that there were new types of MRI scanning that could complement the biopsy result and make active surveillance safer.

Mr Cohen asked for a referral to a specialist who was known to be more comfortable with active surveillance and chose active surveillance in the end, thus avoiding all the discomfort, risks and complications of surgery and he remained well for two years without evidence of progression. He was aware of the fact that about 30% of patients on active surveillance may eventually need surgery but, even if eventually he became one of those patients requiring surgery, at least he would have reduced the length of his life that was affected by the consequences of a prostatectomy.

Xu has described how the decision-making process, in men diagnosed with prostate cancer, was affected by how the information about the prostate cancer diagnosis was processed at two levels:[14]

a) **The affective level: fear of cancer and death** led many men to want it "taken out" with surgery and as soon as possible regardless of any possible side-effects of surgery. This fear could possibly not be fully justified in this cohort of men almost all with Gleason 6 and low risk: active surveillance would have been fully acceptable for many of them, but Xu reported that few recalled having been told about active surveillance.

b) **The cognitive level:** rational weighing of pros and cons of a specific treatment option.

Should urologist put more emphasis, at the time of diagnosis, on the fact that in most cases there is no great urgency to decide? Prostate cancer has a slow progression, hence there is time to ponder and make the right decision that suits each individual.

So, has there been an "invasion of the Prostate Snatchers"?

This is the catchy title of the book written by Blum and Scholz.[4] The main theme in this book is that too many biopsies and too much treatment (prostatectomies in particular, but radiotherapy as well) have been administered to patients with elevated PSA, and this has happened on quite a large scale in the USA, as it was driven by the implementation of PSA screening. In essence the authors argue for more targeted use of prostatic biopsies and for more frequent use of active surveillance as opposed to active treatment. In 2012 the US Preventive Task Force issued new guidance on prostate cancer screening and recommended that PSA-based screening should no longer be used, on the basis of an analysis of benefits and harms of screening.[15] One of the harms of screening is clearly overtreatment and a subsequently published analysis by Jacobs of prostate cancer patients in the USA showed that in 2004–09 there was large scale use of surgical or radiotherapy treatment in those groups of patients who are least likely to benefit, such as men with low-risk disease for whom arguably active surveillance is often a better option, and men with a high-risk of non-cancer mortality.[16] The question is why this is happening. Are there perverse financial incentives? Are urologist and radiotherapists just keen on reducing uncertainty, about progression or undergrading, or just overenthusiastic in plying their trade? Are patients unable to exercise informed choice or just overwhelmed by anxiety? The argument of Richard Blum is that the diagnosis process of a prostate cancer, with the wording used and the limited time for information, all contribute to transform the patient into a *dutiful lamb being herded into the pen* of either prostatectomy or radiotherapy.[4] Blum was a Gleason 7 (3+4) prostate cancer patient who chose active surveillance with apparent good results and better quality of life: some active surveillance studies have included some Gleason 7 (3+4) patients and the new MRI methodologies may allow better monitoring. Is this the direction of march?

Similarly, Xu reported that American men diagnosed with prostate cancer even in recent times were often not told about the option of active surveillance, and that fear of cancer progression and death was often a major contributor to rushed decision making.[14]

Jay Cohen argues in his book that discouraging screening was a retrograde step and that the benefits versus harms balance can be changed, not just by increasing the number of patients on active surveillance, but also by adopting new technologies like the DCE-MRI (or multiparametric MRI) that may allow a reduction in the number of biopsies, better targeted biopsies and safer monitoring of patients on active surveillance.[5] Multiparametric MRI is known to have high sensitivity for the detection of clinically significant prostate cancers (larger cancers and/or grades 7 and above) and can detect cancers missed by the commonly performed random biopsies: thus when there is suspicion of prostate cancer, in spite of negative biopsies, MRI-targeted biopsies are recommended.[17] But prostate biopsies are unpleasant and carry some risks: why take a chance with blind biopsies missing a suspected prostate cancer? There are other advantages with multiparametric MRI: it improves the accuracy of staging,[18] and by guiding the biopsies it reduces the risk not only of missing cancer but also of underestimating the aggressiveness (giving an incorrect lower Gleason grade) by not targeting the most important lesion.[19]

Choosing the treatment modality

There are quite a few websites with information about prostate cancer treatment including the sites from Prostate Cancer Foundation (USA) and Prostate Cancer UK. Personally, I found the book written by Dr Chodak extremely useful: for each treatment modality (and there are quite a few) there is discussion of who is a good candidate for that modality, as well as pros and cons.[2] Chapter 17 of this book is a recap of the options for clinically localised prostate cancer and the Table in that chapter is a very good summary of key considerations. Chapter 16 and Table 16.2 are also very good at helping to make up one's mind.

It is very difficult to go to an appointment with a specialist to decide your treatment modalities, unless you have already done a bit of reading yourself and defined what questions you would like to ask. As Alan Lawrenson says in his book: *you will find that your medical team can only spend limited time with you at each stage… you cannot possibly ask all the right questions and get sufficient information from your doctors.*[8] In essence what Alan Lawrenson says, and I would agree, is that you need to arm yourself with as much information as possible before you see your specialist, so that there can be a more informed discussion. Others have commented that the medical consultation time is by necessity time-defined *thus limiting the amount of time to assess just how much the patient has understood about their prostate cancer diagnosis… for patients with prostate cancer who are faced with a multitude of management options, a high degree of sophistication is required to understand the nuanced details of different options* (see chapter 16 of this reference textbook).[3] A significant degree of health literacy is required and a willingness to self-educate: health literacy can make a real difference to outcomes and probably explains some of the outcomes inequalities across different social classes.

Some very important initial considerations are your age and general level of health. The older you are and the more medical conditions you have, the higher the surgical risks are and the balance may shift towards the radiotherapy options (of which there are a few). Radiotherapy may carry a small risk of secondary bladder and rectal cancer, but the risk decreases if you have a shorter life expectancy. Having read Dr Chodak's book, I decided that androgen-deprivation therapy was the treatment modality I most disliked (and not really suitable as the initial treatment modality at my age). Looking at Table 16.2 of Dr Chodak's book,[2] I felt I disliked radical prostatectomy less than I disliked radiotherapy: I have ulcerative colitis (though well controlled) thus I was more worried about the radiation side-effects (problems with the bowel) than the side-effects of the prostatectomy. Many of us would perhaps like to choose the treatment that is most effective and least likely to be followed by a relapse: however, as Dr Chodak says,[2] there are no long-term studies comparing efficacy. In essence the choice (as far as I can see it) is more about which side-effects of each treatment we dislike less, rather than efficacy. An argument used by surgeons in favour of prostatectomy is that, if you have a relapse, you might still be able to have radiotherapy as a rescue strategy, vice versa if you relapse after radiotherapy surgery would be difficult. In my case I felt surgery fitted better with my outlook on life. Prostatectomy is a major procedure: surely it takes time to recover, but the consequences such as urinary incontinence or erectile dysfunction tend to improve or even resolve with time. With radiotherapy you are never admitted to hospital and you do not have to recover from a major procedure, but there seem to be more long-lasting side-effects and the small risk of a bladder/colorectal cancer after 10 or more years. However, if I had been older and frailer I would have probably gone for radiotherapy. If you decide to have radiotherapy, you need to define the precise modality and find out whether concurrent androgen-deprivation therapy, usually for a limited period of time, is also required.

If you are inclined to go for a prostatectomy, there two other important issues that need to be discussed and clarified:

- Is it possible to spare the neurovascular bundles on one or both sides? If so, you are less likely to suffer from erectile dysfunction and incontinence, but the risk of a cancer relapse is higher if you are thought to have a higher risk of extracapsular extension.
- Can the lymph nodes be left alone or does the surgeon recommend a lymph node dissection? The lymph node dissection prolongs the surgical procedure and increases the risk of side-effects, but it might reduce the risk of relapses. You can see a discussion of the pros and cons of lymph node dissection in chapter 10 of Dr Chodak's book[2] and in these articles.[20, 21] The European Guidelines on prostate cancer recommend an extended lymph node dissection when the risk of lymph node involvement is above 5%:[17] there are various nomograms to calculate the risk of lymph node involvement, but the Briganti nomogram seems to be the best.[22]

While you have to consider the advice given to you, your views and attitudes also matter. When the risk of relapse is low, most men would prefer a nerve-sparing procedure without excision of the lymph nodes. Surprisingly, though, according to Jay Cohen, some surgeons appear to recommend removal of the neurovascular bundles even in low-risk patients with Gleason 6 grade cancer when a less aggressive approach or even active surveillance might be preferable options.[5] If you know precisely what surgical option is offered to you, then you might be able to reconsider your choices: for instance you may prefer surgery over radiotherapy, but if you are told that you need removal of both nerve bundles and the lymph nodes, maybe you may now think you want to reconsider radiotherapy.

Not everybody feels confident enough to choose a treatment modality and many would prefer the specialist to make the choice for them. You might feel that dealing with the emotional side of having been diagnosed with cancer is bad enough, and that you would rather leave the "technical side" to the specialist. Some might also feel that asking for a second opinion or a reflection pause might delay surgery, when they actually they want to "get it out" as soon as possible. In most prostate cancer cases there is no great urgency for the surgical procedure, but psychologically one might feel better only after the procedure.

Prostate cancer survivors who have written books about their cancer journey tend to be different beasts: they usually like to seek information from various sources and other specialists before making up their mind and expressing their preferences. Mr Lawrenson perhaps did a more extensive search than most of the other book authors: the first specialist he met recommended either prostatectomy or radiotherapy, but after that he sought a second and third opinion from two other urologist practising High-Intensity Focused Ultrasound (HIFU).[8] As neither recommended this treatment for him, he then did a temporary procedure to improve the urinary obstruction (TURP) and started androgen deprivation treatment; finally he decided to undergo proton beam radiation but, as it was not available in Australia where he lived, he travelled to South Korea for that.[8]

Not many of us would make the same choice in terms of seeking treatment in a faraway country at a significant cost. Dr Chodak in his book makes negative comments about proton beam radiation: *no study has yet shown either better results or fewer side effects... actually, two recent nonrandomised studies have found more side effects with PBR compared with conventional radiation.*[2] But, on the other side, being able to get the type of treatment you think is best for you is morale uplifting. In general, scanning the literature for new diagnostic or treatment modalities can be advantageous: when new methodologies giving better results are introduced, uptake of the new procedure or diagnostic test may be slow (for all sorts of reasons including cost): sometimes it pays to go to a different regional or national centre. I chose the hospital where I have been treated because they were more willing to use MRI as a diagnostic tool, and I believe I benefitted from better targeted biopsies.

I think the advice Dr Chodak gives in his book about choosing a treatment modality is solid,[2] treatment depends on: *your age, health, and tumour properties. But equally important is the need to factor in your personal goals and fears and your personality type… your personality should be an important part of choosing your therapy.* Another reason why your preferences should matter, according to Dr Chodak, is that: *although many doctors have strong opinions about which treatment is best, the truth is that no one knows for sure because optimal studies have not been done.*[2] When two or more treatment options are roughly equivalent, but carry different risks and disadvantages, then there is some scope for personal choice. In the decision process, I would bear in mind the saying: "a little knowledge is a dangerous thing". You may decide to ignore the recommendation of one specialist, but it might be unwise to ignore the recommendations of all the specialists.

Chodak advises to involve your partner (this is often conducive to more balanced decisions) and to talk to other patients.[2] Many men have reported that the experience of other men they knew was influential: these men could be celebrities reported in the media or friends.[14] For instance one of the men interviewed by Xu, who eventually decided to have radiotherapy, said: A *good friend of mine had surgery. He was a young man going in and he has nothing now. He dribbles, he's incontinent, and he doesn't have sexual function. I couldn't imagine myself in that way.*[14] Personally I would be cautious here, talking to other men who have undergone treatment is extremely important and useful, but we could draw wrong conclusions from a sample of one man talking to us, when large published reports of the outcomes of that procedure might paint a different picture. Alan Lawrenson for instance, in his book about his experience as a prostate cancer patient reports that, although brachytherapy had been recommended as a suitable treatment for him, he refused to consider this option because: *my sample of one person (my brother) undergoing this type of treatment had shown a recurrence of the cancer eight years later.*[8] Perhaps one could have kept brachytherapy in the short-list and could have assessed the comparative pros and cons on the basis of the reported results from large groups of patients.

Many patients do not feel confident or competent in making their own choices, whilst others may have very set ideas regarding how they want to be treated. There is also an intermediate option: you may not know precisely what treatment is best for you, but you know what side-effects you fear most and what your life goals are. So, if you are younger and having a sex life is important and you are prepared to take slightly higher risk of relapse, speak to your specialist as it might steer you towards either nerve-sparing surgery or radiotherapy. Conversely if you have been troubled by ulcerative colitis and fear having even more severe bowel symptoms, voice your concerns as it might direct your specialist to recommend surgery. And if you felt that length of life is the most important thing, more than quality, say that as they may offer you the more aggressive options if you are prepared to take the risk of the side-effects.

Getting a second opinion

Annette Bloch in her book recalls how her father in 1978 was diagnosed with lung cancer and given three month to live, but they sought a second opinion, he underwent a difficult treatment and was cured to live another 26 years.[23] A second opinion could be valuable even in less extreme circumstances.

For me prostate cancer treatment has been the most important decision about my health, so far in my life. I am sure this would be the case for many others. Well worthwhile getting a second opinion! So, if you have met with a surgeon who has proposed a prostatectomy, why not get an appointment with a radiation oncologist to hear what the radio-therapy options would be. Conversely if like me, you are happy with a surgeon proposing a prostatectomy but hesitate about some of the details (nerve-sparing or not, lymph node dissection or not) or you are worried about the side effects or the risk of relapse, why not to ask your family doctor to refer you to another prostate surgeon in a differ-ent hospital; it might also be an opportunity to compare the caseload or the experience or the interpersonal skills of the two surgeons.

Sometimes the second opinion can change the course of your life! Lawrenson in his book reports the case of a 55-year-old man with advanced prostate cancer who had been treated with androgen-depri-vation therapy, but had become unresponsive to this treatment; he hesitated about the proposal to undertake chemotherapy and asked for a referral to a different specialist, who was able to get a treatment response without resorting to chemotherapy.[8] Similarly Jay Cohen had been offered an aggressive prostatectomy, but the second specialist he contacted was happy to have him on active surveillance.[5]

The attitude towards seeking a second opinion seems to vary signifi-cantly in different surveys. Some previous reports based mostly on men attending urology clinics appeared to suggest that few men sought a second opinion; however, a more recent survey of American patients recruited from both urology and radiation oncology centres showed that most men (17 out of 21 men interviewed) had sought at least one second professional opinion.[14] This survey captured two atti-tudes in relation to seeking a second professional opinion:

- Four men did not want a second opinion because of a concern about delaying treatment, or because of perceiving difficulties with receiving a second opinion and then having to decide between conflicting advice, or because they felt they had trust in their urologist or in God.
- 17 men choose to have a second/third opinion from either another urologist or a radiation oncologist or from their family doctor or even a physician acquaintance: seeking further professional opinions was problematic because the

42

second opinion frequently conflicted with the first, and this could cause confusion and anxiety. Thus, seeking a second opinion would fit better a self-reliant personality with willingness to weigh pros and cons and to make the final choice.

Trust or distrust of the first specialist doctor can be an important determinant in seeking a second opinion. Xu reported that black men in particular felt distrust of physicians and the healthcare system: one man even questioned whether there were financial motivations behind a recommendation of "unnecessary surgery" whereas another one felt he had more confidence in his doctor because he was a black man.[14]

Looking up a discussion thread on a UK Prostate Cancer website, it seems that some centres routinely offer the opportunity of meeting both a urology surgeon and a radiation oncologist (either simultaneously or sequentially) and some patients are routinely offered a range of treatment options suitable for their circumstances, with built-in time for the patient to learn and reflect before a final decision is expected.

Choosing a surgeon

Not all hospitals offer prostate cancer surgery or radiotherapy. You can usually work out from various websites which are the centres and who are the specialists working there. But who are the best specialists, or at least those with the greatest experience? It is not easy to answer this question, but what you can do is:

- Check the online profile of each specialist, their areas of interest and any reference to caseload.
- You can use Google Scholar Author Search to see which specialist has scientific/medical publications, although academic talent is not synonymous with clinical skills.
- Word of mouth: do you know any healthcare workers working in the same hospital? Or do you know any patients treated by them? Go to local support group meetings.

- If you decide to have a prostatectomy, caseload and experience are conducive to better results. Chodak recommends choosing a surgeon who does more than 20–40 prostatectomies per year.[2] When you see your specialist, do not be afraid to ask how many they have done in their whole career and how many they currently do each year. Surgeons may not volunteer this information, but if asked they are meant to give an honest answer. And if you are going for a "robotic prostatectomy", you must ask for the caseload limited to that procedure, robotic prostatectomy being very different from open prostatectomy.

Jay Cohen makes another quite important and pertinent recommendation: *Most important in making your decision to have prostate surgery is to find a urologic surgeon you trust. In addition to having extensive experience with the technique being used, this surgeon should be willing to patiently and fully answer all your questions.*[5]

Risk of secondary cancers after radiotherapy

This is a particular risk that I have not seen discussed in Dr Chodak's book, but that might play a role in deciding which treatment to go for. We have known for some time that exposure to radiation increases the risk of cancer, but quantifying the risk is very difficult because radiotherapy modalities change all the time and you need very long term studies (10–20 years) to assess this risk. We know that the risk is greater in younger patients and this may reflect both a greater susceptibility and a longer lifespan during which secondary tumours may occur. The website of the American Cancer Society has some generic information on the risk of secondary cancers, which is not specific for prostate cancer radiotherapy, and that can be summarised as follows:

- Increased risk of bone marrow malignancy such as leukemias: peak incidence is five to nine years after exposure, age at which exposure occurs does not seem to matter.
- Solid tumours such as colorectal or bladder cancers: mostly occur 10–15 years after the exposure, age of exposure matters with lower risk later in life.

44

However which part of the body is treated can make a big difference, hence we need to look at secondary cancer risk data which are specific for the radiotherapy of prostate cancer.

The best summary for the risks of secondary cancers after radiotherapy of prostate cancers seems to be in a recent review article which concluded that there was an increased risk of either bladder or colorectal cancers (but not bone marrow malignancies) but only after external radiotherapy and not after brachytherapy.[24] However, the absolute difference in the risk of cancer between those treated with radiotherapy, and those not treated with this modality, was small: up to 0.6% for bladder cancers and up to 1.4% for colorectal cancers.[24] I presume that if the studies reviewed in this article had been extended over a longer period of time the overall risk, though probably still small, might have increased. The authors of this review article concluded with a recommendation that appears sensible: *In particular, for patients with a long life expectancy of 20 years or more, the possibility of secondary malignancy related to radiation needs to be included in management discussion.*[24]

Prostatectomy day: the phoney war is over

At the beginning of World War II, after the UK and France declared war on Germany on 3 September 1939, not much happened on the western front for about eight months. It was surreal: another major conflict had started (just 21 years after the end of World War I) but not much was happening.

I felt the same. I had an outpatient appointment on 29 September 2016 during which I was told the histology of my prostate biopsies had shown I had cancer. My prostatectomy took place on 24 October 2016. Between these two dates not much happened apart from the pre-surgical assessment. And the fact was, I was perfectly well, no symptoms attributable to prostate cancer. It felt surreal. I sometimes wondered whether it was not just a bad dream.

It is difficult to accept that you have cancer and you need a major surgical procedure when you are perfectly well. This is not however a unique situation, it can happen to women as well: they might be perfectly well but a screening mammogram may show a lesion that turns out to be breast cancer.

Sometimes things have to get worse before they get better.

Sick leave after a prostatectomy

If you are still at work, when you undergo a prostatectomy, you will need to take a period of sick leave. So, what shall you tell your boss or your colleagues or what plan should you make for yourself if you are self-employed? The hospital stay is usually short (just above 48 hours in my case), but what about the length of your sick leave?

A friend of mine told me he had been at home for about three months: but he had done an open prostatectomy (radical retropubic prostatectomy, not a robotic one) and had suffered from a leg deep vein thrombosis: both events would have extended his recovery time.

My urology consultant told me I should expect a period of six weeks sick leave to recover at home, as prostatectomy is a major procedure and you need to work on your recovery. I was told to continue the venous embolism prophylaxis for a total of four weeks. The robotic prostatectomy leaflet, issued to me by the hospital before the surgical procedure, emphasised these points about my road to fitness strategy:

- Continue wearing anti-embolic stockings and daily subcutaneous injections of tinzaparin for four weeks.
- Find time (after the catheter removal) for the pelvic exercises in order to facilitate the return of urinary continence.
- Exercise beginning with gentle exercises such as walking for 15 minutes (verbally I had been told to do only light exercises with no stress on the abdomen for eight weeks).
- Do not drive for at least two weeks and until you are confident you can control the car.
- Do not return to your normal routine for at least four weeks and expect to return to work about six weeks after the surgical procedure.

When I phoned my family doctor the day after my hospital discharge, he sent me a six weeks sick note for my employer.

There are only two recent medical publications on the length of sick leave, that I could retrieve via a Medline (medical literature) search. The most recent one is a Norwegian study: this included patients undergoing both the old-style "open" retropubic prostatectomy and robotic prostatectomy.[25] The introduction mentions the fact that Norwegian urologists routinely prescribe four to six weeks of sick leave (with a possibility of an extension prescribed by the family doctor), whereas Swedish guidelines recommend six weeks of sick leave. The key findings in this study were that 51% of the patients had returned to work six weeks after the prostatectomy and 66% after seven to eight weeks, but 27% were still on part or full-time sick leave after 10 weeks. A number of factors were associated with a longer time to return to work: such as doing a physically demanding work and having had an "open" prostatectomy rather than a robotic one. The authors also assessed "declined" work status three months after the prostatectomy: in other words, they looked at what proportion of the men were still on sick leave or had left work or had moved from full-time to part-time work. There was a tendency for patients experiencing moderate or severe urinary continence problems being more likely to have "declined" work status (but no conclusive statistical evidence for this observation). The main finding was that a reduction in the physical well-being after surgery, measured through compilation of a questionnaire, was the only factor with a statistically significant association with "declined" work status. Thus, regaining general physical fitness, and possibly urinary continence, seem to be the determining factors for a return to work.

The other article I have retrieved showed a much shorter period of sick leave for robotic prostatectomy (11 days) as opposed to open prostatectomy (49 days).[26] There are issues with this article. First of all, did "11 days" mean 11 working days, which is just about more than two weeks if you work Monday–Friday? Secondly it seems that the patients undergoing the robotic prostatectomy were fitter (hence a somewhat shorter period of sick leave might be expected) and that the doctors might have been biased by offering shorter sick leave to patients undergoing the robotic prostatectomy. In my experience, though, proper full work after two weeks is unrealistic.

I think most of us will know when we are ready to go back to work and maybe a gradual/phased resumption of work activities is a better option.

Risk of hernia after a robotic prostatectomy

An incisional hernia is a protrusion of the intra-abdominal tissues (which may include bowel loops) through the surgical incision sites (in this case the port hole cuts) due to incomplete healing of the surgical wound. It manifests with the appearance of a bulge that can be painful. The risk of incisional hernia seems to be greater with laparoscopic or robotic prostatectomies than with open prostatectomies and the risk is higher in those with a previous history of hernia repair.[27]

Inguinal hernias (hernias in the groin and not at any of the surgical port sites) may also appear after a prostatectomy procedure: the risk seems to increase with age, lower body weight and a previous history of inguinal hernia repair.[28] This might be one of the few situations in which obesity is actually a benefit.

There does not seem to be much that we can do to reduce the risk of either incision or inguinal hernia other than reporting any previous hernia history when discussing treatment modalities, as it may have an impact on the choice of surgical procedure or its modalities. Good nutrition and minimising the risk of haematoma and infection at the port sites might help.

Risk of deep vein thrombosis (DVT) after a robotic prostatectomy

A deep vein thrombosis (DVT) is a blood clot in a vein, most frequently in the legs and especially in the calves. The typical symptoms are pain, tenderness and swelling. Pulmonary embolus (migration of a clot piece to the lungs) is a feared complication, and it would manifest with chest pain, cough and shortness of breath. Pulmonary embolism is serious and can lead to death. It is important to have a timely diagnosis of DVT to allow appropriate treatment. The risk of either DVT or pulmonary embolism is increased in these groups of patients: patients undergoing lymph node dissection together with the prostatectomy, patients with a previous history of DVT or pulmonary embolism,[29] current smokers, patients who have to go back to theatre for a second surgical procedure, and in patients with either a longer operative time or a longer hospital stay.[30] Some surgeons may argue that low risk patients may not require the administration of anticoagulants like heparin as a preventative strategy.[30] In patients undergoing lymph node dissection the greatest risk is between day 14 and day 28 postoperatively, thus prophylactic measures might be beneficial for four weeks.[29]

The risk of surgical patients developing DVT can be reduced with the use of compression stockings and thromboprophylaxis (giving anticoagulants with the aim of preventing thrombosis). After my robotic prostatectomy, I was told to wear the anti-embolism stockings and inject myself subcutaneously with tinzaparin sodium (a type of anticoagulant) for four weeks. There may be differences in practice in the use of anticoagulant prophylaxis between different countries, for instance a survey in 2004 found that only 24% of the urologists in the USA used anticoagulant prophylaxis as opposed to 100% of the British urologists.[31]

In addition to anti-embolism stockings and anticoagulants, there are other things we can do to further reduce the risk of DVT:

- Drinking plenty of fluids: dehydration increases the risk.
- Avoiding immobility of the legs: for instance, walking as much as possible at regular intervals (do not sit for too long).
- Stopping smoking before a prostatectomy.

If you, like me, have had to wear anti-embolism stockings over a period of four weeks, you will have put them on and taken them off many times. You will have noticed the strengthened area that goes over the heel. And you may have asked yourself why do these stockings need to have a hole that goes over the plantar side of the foot and the toes, and always end-up in the wrong place? The hole is an "inspection hole" useful if you are an inpatient requiring a check on the perfusion of the feet, but just useless when you have left the hospital.

Penile rehabilitation after a prostatectomy

When I re-attended the hospital one week after the nerve-sparing prostatectomy, my catheter was removed and I was prescribed sildenafil (Viagra) 50mg every other day for six months. A study published in 2008 has shown that recovery of erectile function after nerve-sparing prostatectomy is faster if treatment with sildenafil (25mg at night) starts on the day of the catheter removal: peak recovery was one year after surgery.[32] Conversely a second study showed that sildenafil on demand (when sexual activity was undertaken) was as good as sildenafil daily.[33] The concept of penile rehabilitation is discussed in greater detail in chapter 62 of the reference textbook:[3] other medications have been used for penile rehabilitation including alprostadil used either in the intraurethal format (a small pellet inserted in the urethra) or the intracavernosal format (penile injection).

I got the impression that early sexual intercourse supported by erectile dysfunction medications might be as good as daily sildenafil. This is probably just another example of "use it or lose it". There are comments on this topic in the website of the James Buchanan Brady Urological Institute, the institution where one of the studies was conducted http://urology.jhu.edu/newsletter/2014/prostate_cancer_2014_6.php

Treatment for erectile dysfunction after prostatectomy is discussed on these websites:

http://prostatecanceruk.org/prostate-information/living-with-prostate-cancer/sex-and-relationships

http://www.ustoo.org/PDFs/Manage_Impotence.pdf

An alternative (or complementary) strategy for penile rehabilitation is the use of vacuum devices: these devices consists of pumps attached to plastic cylinders, which create a vacuum around the penis thus making blood flow into it to make it hard. In one study based on the use of these devices, starting one month after the prostatectomy gave better results than starting after six months.[34] Early use of the vacuum pump also reduced the penile length loss which follows the prostatectomy.[34]

This comment in chapter 62 of the reference textbook summarises some of the uncertainties regarding the optimal strategy for penile rehabilitation: *although penile rehabilitation is widely accepted, a consensus or optimal strategy has yet to be determined*.[3]

Pelvic floor muscles (Kegel) exercises

Weeks before my prostatectomy procedure, I had been given the instructions for these exercises, which are meant to improve the post-surgical urinary continence. The bit that I found difficult in the instruction sheets was where it said: *try not to squeeze your buttocks together or tighten your abdominal muscles*. I cannot do these exercises without squeezing at least the buttocks, at least in part. Does it really matter?

However, the main question I asked myself was: are these exercises just a fad, or are they really useful?

There are studies suggesting that pelvic floor exercises can speed up the recovery of continence[35] and starting the pelvic floor exercises before the surgical procedure might be advantageous.[36] However, in the long term most men will recover continence even without pelvic floor exercises: thus 12 months after the prostatectomy there is not much difference between those who did the exercises and those who did not (see chapter 32 of the reference book).[3]

So, what is my personal take on this? I am a gym man and I am biased towards exercising. And, doing something to help myself fits well with the fighting spirit approach. Although the advantage of the exercises seems to be mostly limited to the first 12 months after surgery, getting a bit more continence a bit earlier can boost morale.

Now, I must confess, I did not start the exercises before the prostatectomy, although I went once weekly to either a Pilates or a yoga class, which might also strengthen the pelvic floor muscles. So, depending on whether I keep doing or not the pelvic floor muscles exercises, my probability of achieving continence at various intervals post-surgery seems to be as by the Table 2. At one and three months post-surgery more than twice as many men achieved continence with the exercises than without. After 12 months there was a smaller difference, still in favour of doing the exercises but this difference was not statistically significant (in other words with this sample size it is not possible to prove that the small advantage after 12 months is real).

Table 2. Percentage of men achieving continence (defined as either "completely dry" or "occasional leakage") at various intervals after a prostatectomy with or without pelvic floor muscle exercises.[35]

pelvic floor muscle exercises	1 month	3 months	6 months	12 months
YES	19.3%	74.0%	96.0%	98.7%
NO	8.0%	30.0%	64.6%	88.0%

But do the above benefits from the exercises really apply to me? In the clinical trial from which these data come, the patients assigned to the pelvic floor exercises were given three training sessions and were also encouraged to count the episodes of urinary leakage and to increase the frequency of micturition if they experienced leakages. It is possible that exercises learnt from written instructions may not be learnt properly, and the motivation to sustain the use of the exercises might be less strong.

On the issue of recovering continence more quickly, the written instructions given to me recommended to cut down the intake of any drinks containing caffeine: these include tea, coffee, cocoa and cola. The reason for this recommendation is the reported association between caffeine intake and urinary incontinence symptoms. Caffeine, however, is also a central nervous system stimulant: thus, most of us drink caffeinated beverages to control tiredness or fatigue during our day at work. Personally, I am quite dependent on caffeine to keep going mentally, but I have noticed the worsening of stress incontinence after caffeinated drinks. Is there an alternative to caffeine?

Obviously, there are decaffeinated versions of tea and coffee: a friend of mine has suggested she can fool her brain and get mental stimulation even from the decaffeinated drinks. Alternatively, I might try ginseng tea, allegedly it is also a mental stimulant but without impact on bladder activity, although I have not seen any hard evidence for either of these claims.

An interesting finding from one of these studies is that men who had a nerve-sparing prostatectomy had better continence.[35] In some of the reference sources nerve-sparing is presented as a less invasive procedure that allows a higher probability of retaining erectile function, but this and some other studies suggest that there may also be an advantage in terms of urinary continence. This is an important issue to discuss with your urology surgeon before the prostatectomy: nerve-sparing may carry a higher risk of not removing the prostate cancer entirely, particularly when there are reasons to believe it has already extended outside the prostate's capsule.

A minority of patients may still have severe urinary continence problems even months after the procedure. If this happens, you need to be aware of the fact that there are other things that could be tried, the list includes electrical muscle stimulation, specific medications and specific surgical procedures: see chapter 18 of Dr Chodak's book[2] or chapter 32 of the reference book.[3] In essence instead of giving up, you could ask for an appointment with a specialist to discuss the options.

Continence pads

You have had a prostatectomy. Welcome to the world of continence pads. You will need pads, at least for the initial period. For many men, this is a new experience. What can I say about this? Walk to your local supermarket: there is a range of brands and a range of products marketed for men. The smaller pads are less obtrusive and more comfortable, but have more limited capacity to absorb. The larger ones are uncomfortable and may force you to buy larger trousers.

The thing is, I have not yet found a really perfect type of pad! I have not needed a large absorbance capacity: yes, I have suffered from multiple leaks in a day (more in the afternoon and evening than in the morning and usually none during the night) but all small volume leaks. Thus, I tend to use the smaller triangular shaped pads, quite adequate in absorbance capacity, but not in "coverage" and this despite my efforts at really careful positioning inside the pants. Couldn't these pads come in a range of sizes, or just be a bit wider?

The average flaccid penis is about 9 cm in length: beware! The penis can go in any direction covering the full 360° circle. For instance, I may position mine in the upright position, but on standing or walking it falls on either side and then goes "out of range" as demonstrated in Figure 2 with the *Tena Men level 2* pads. The consequence of going out of range are that you wet your pants, if not your trousers as well. Obviously there has been a need to change strategy. I have experimented with the *Boots Staydry for Men Extra*: unfortunately, they are precisely the same size and shape, but they have elasticated straps on the sides though, honestly, these straps could be a bit wider. Thus, my new strategy (Figure 3) is:

a) position the pad a bit further down in the pants (especially during daytime), I am giving up upright coverage but, during daytime gravity makes this unnecessary;
b) tuck my penis inside the side strap;
c) use reasonably tight pants.

The new strategy works better, though it is always prudent to have spare pads and pants at hand (just in case). There is another strategy to maximise tightness and reduce the risk of leaks: you can wear your pad inside a fixation pant like the Tena fix, and then put your regular pants on top. Yes, it does seem to reduce the risk of leaks, but I do not like it: it feels too tight and hot. Like many men, I like to keep things down there a bit loose and cool.

Having incontinence can be quite demoralising. But there is a range of strategies we can use to define the problem, minimise the impact and speed up the recovery.

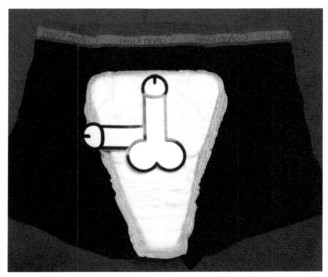

Figure 2. My experience with the *Tena Men level 2* pads: if the penis is positioned upright, this pad is not wide enough as, when the penis falls sideways, "it goes out of range" and you wet your pants.

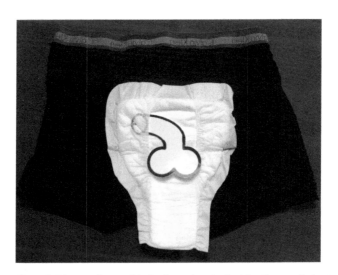

Figure 3. My experience with the *Boots Staydry for Men Extra* pads: best results are achieved by positioning the pad a bit further down to maximise lateral and lower coverage. Tucking your penis in one of the straps helps to keep it inside and "in range". Wider elasticated bands would be better.

Urinary Tract Infection

Urinary Tract Infections (UTIs) are uncommon in men younger than 50. Some UTIs in men are due to or facilitated by prostate conditions, such as prostatitis and benign prostate hyperplasia. After a prostatectomy UTIs can occur, initially because of the catheter insertion, and later on because the prostate removal has disrupted some of the protective barriers. Bacteria are often present in the distal urethra and the groin area: infections are due to bacteria migrating further up the urinary system against the urinary flow.

The typical symptoms of UTIs are:

- pain when passing urine;
- need to pass urine more frequently;
- fever (not always present).

Diagnosing a UTI just after a prostatectomy is more difficult as both pain in passing urine and frequency might also be a consequence of the surgical procedure. There are urine tests that, if positive, make the diagnosis of UTI more likely:

- Urine dipsticks. These are strips with little pads to detect various analytes and give an immediate result: the presence of nitrite or leukocyte may indicate infection.
- Urine culture. This takes two to three days and the presence of bacteria may indicate infection. Any bacteria present are usually tested to identify which antibiotics might be appropriate (antibiotic sensitivity test).

When symptoms and/or the rapid dipstick test suggest a UTI, antibiotics are usually started (empirical treatment): there is no certainty at this stage that the antibiotics are appropriate. If a urine culture has been requested, antibiotic sensitivity testing of any bacteria detected in the urine will confirm (or not) whether the chosen antibiotic is appropriate.

Patients who have not responded to treatment (and have persisting symptoms) could go back to see their family doctor two to three days later: at this stage, there should be a culture result with antibiotic sensitivity testing results.

Patients who develop SEPSIS must attend an urgent care centre as a matter of urgency: sepsis is a severe infection that can arise from different body sites, including the urinary tract, and can be life-threatening. Most UTIs are not associated with sepsis, but some are. After a surgical procedure sepsis can also occur as a result of infection at the surgical site. The UK Sepsis Trust recommends that patients seek urgent medical advice if they develop any of these:

- **S**lurred speech.
- **E**xtreme shivering or muscle pain.
- **P**assing no urine (in a day).
- **S**evere breathlessness.
- **I** feel like I might die.
- **S**kin mottled or discoloured.

Information on sepsis is also available from the CDC website in the USA: https://www.cdc.gov/sepsis/basic/qa.html

Preventing Urinary Tract Infections while you are catheterised

After a prostatectomy, many patients are discharged home with a catheter and must look after the catheter. Verbal or written instructions will be given, but of variable quality. There is a guideline document, that summarises the key points in preventing the acquisition of an infection from catheters, which can be downloaded from the CDC website.[37] The key thing to remember is that the drainage system is intended to have a one-way flow from your bladder down to the collection bag. Bacteria may multiply inside the collection system and bag, and you do not want the urine from the collection bag to flow back into your bladder! Thus, make sure that:

- You maintain an unobstructed urine flow: keep the catheter and collecting tube free from kinking.
- You empty the collecting bag regularly (wash hands before and after).

- You keep the collecting bag BELOW the level of the bladder at all times (or else the urine might flow back). Do not rest the bag on the floor, use a stand.

Diet and supplements: do they make a difference?

There are three aspects of the diet that needs to be discussed. Firstly, can we change our diet to reduce the risk of developing prostate cancer? Secondly, can diet help AFTER we have been diagnosed with prostate cancer? Thirdly, are food supplements helpful and which ones?

The answer to the first question seems to be that diet is probably a MODIFIABLE risk factor for prostate cancer: and I write modifiable in capital letters! There are other risk factors such as age or having an immediate family member with prostate cancer, but there is nothing we can do about these risk factors. The identification of diet as a risk factor is partially based on the observation that prostate cancer is less common in some Asian countries, and that migrants from those countries adopting western diets are no longer protected, but it is really difficult to know for sure which foods are the good ones and which are the bad ones. There is some experimental work suggesting some foods have anti-cancer properties, but it is always very difficult to extrapolate from experimental work, and the effect in real life may not be substantial or significant. There are also epidemiological studies based on food consumption questionnaires in individuals with or without prostate cancer: but what we eat is something we change all the time and, this is the bottom line, epidemiological studies can find associations but cannot prove causality in a definitive way, even when there is adjustment for possible confounders. *The Prostate Care Cookbook* published in association with the Prostate Cancer Research Foundation seems to be a good book, and I found it to be a very good source of information.[38] In fact, I found it so useful that I bought two extra copies, one for each of my sons, in the hope that a healthy diet could compensate the risk of having a father with prostate cancer. There are two parts to this book. The introduction explains which foods might decrease or increase the risk of prostate cancer and what is the evidence for this belief (or hypothesis); it also explains how much we may need to eat and whether there are risks from increased consumption. The second part of the book is about recipes with those potentially risk-lowering ingredients: there is no point telling us what is good to eat, if use of those ingredients is alien to our culture or to our time-limited cooking habits. The good foods and bad foods are listed in Table 3.

Table 3. Foods associated with decreased risk of prostate cancer (good) and foods associated with increased risk (bad).	
Good foods	Bad foods (particularly if in excessive amounts)
• Garlic, onions, chives, leeks (better raw than cooked) • Cruciferous vegetables including broccoli, cauliflower, cabbage, Brussels sprouts, rocket, horseradish etc. (better raw than cooked) • Oily fish (containing omega-3 fatty acids and vitamin D): salmon, trout, mackerel, kippers, sardines, tuna (tuna only if fresh and not tinned), anchovies* • Seafood (contains selenium) • Legumes and soya products: beans (including baked beans), peas, lentils, soya milk, tofu etc. • Polyphenols: green tea, pomegranate, raspberries • Lycopene: tomatoes (cooked better than raw), watermelon • Selenium: fish and seafood (avoid brazil nuts and selenium tablets)[3] • Vitamin D: exposure to sun, oily fish, consider vitamin D supplements if living at latitudes above 37 degrees north or below 37 degrees south, as exposure to the sun is inadequate • Vitamin E: nuts, soya beans, chickpeas, parmesan, cheddar cheese, olives, avocados (increase intake via the diet rather than supplements, vitamin E tablets might be harmful)[3]	• Dairy products if in excessive amounts: in the right amount these are important sources of calcium and iodine thus should be consumed in moderation, high intake above "recommended" amount might possibly increase prostate cancer risk • Red meat if in excessive amounts: beef, pork, lamb, goat# • Processed meat: ham, bacon, sausages, salami, Frankfurters (hot dogs)# • Eggs: more than 2.5 per week may increase prostate cancer risk [40, 41] • Poultry with skin: poultry is thought to be a good food but possibly not the skin [40, 41] • Alcohol, particularly excessive consumption[42]
The source for the information in this table is, unless otherwise indicated, the book by Rayman and others.[38] * Pollutants can accumulate in some of these fish, thus the maximum recommended number of portions is four per week # WHO has also issued warning about increased cancer risk in the colon particularly from processed meat and, to a lesser extent, red meat.[39]	

There are similar diet recommendations in documents that can be downloaded from the Prostate Cancer Foundation website[43] and from the Prostate Cancer UK website.[44]

Let me say a few words about processed meats: for a century or two they have been frequently consumed foods in many Western countries including southern European countries like Italy (salami, mortadella, Italian sausage, Parma ham) or northern European/American countries (würstel, frankfurters, sausages, ham, bacon). Processed meats are ingrained in our food tradition and culture. So, when recently the World Health Organisation (WHO) declared that these red processed meats are a carcinogen (for various cancers, it is not just the prostate) an Italian friend of mine told me this was an attack on our culinary culture, and added that he will never give up on processed meats! It made me smile, what is "traditional" about processed meats? Until two or three hundred years ago, most people ate very little meat, cured or not: it was too expensive. As meat consumption started to increase in the 19th century, so did the consumption of processed meats: our forebears did not have a choice, as in the absence of fridges and freezers there was no other way to prevent meat from spoiling. In my parents' generation (Italy in the 1950s and 1960s) processed meats were the obvious and ultimate convenience food: if you came home late and tired and unwilling to cook, all you had to do was to slice your Parma ham or your salami. However, nowadays processed meats no longer serve a useful purpose: we all have fridge and freezers and we can have fresh meat easily all the time, or else any supermarket has plenty of choice of ready to eat healthy convenience foods not based on processed meat. Our "culture" and our way of eating have changed so many times in the past, why not change again on the basis of what is good for us? Many fish or poultry recipes are more delicious than sausages!

Alcohol seems to be a difficult risk factor to assess: previous studies have given conflicting results and some previous review studies have suggested no association between alcohol and prostate cancer risk. However, a new review article, which re-analyses and combines the previous studies, concludes that alcohol consumption might be associated with increased prostate cancer risk and that the risk increases with the amount of alcohol drunk.[42] Readers of this book might start

60

asking: is there anything pleasurable left in life that does not increase the risk of prostate cancer? The problem with this type of epidemiological studies are confounders: so, it is possible that alcohol might appear to be a risk factor just because increasing alcohol drinking is associated with other risk factors such as poor diet or lack of exercise. As the recently published review study[42] shows a dose-response relationship (increased risk with increased drinking), it sounds prudent to avoid excess alcohol drinking (which we may want to do anyway). Keep watching this space.

There are fewer studies that have looked at the influence of diet, after the diagnosis of prostate cancer, on outcomes such as prostate cancer progression (for men on active surveillance) or relapse (after prostatectomy and radiotherapy). It seems prudent to assume that the same foods, which are thought to increase or decrease the risk of prostate cancer, might have the same influence on cancer progression and there is a similar statement in the document by the Prostate Cancer Foundation.[43]

Food supplements

Pantuck and others in 2006 reported on the use of a daily glass of pomegranate juice on men with rising PSA after either surgery or radiation: this research group reported that pomegranate did "appear" to reduce the PSA doubling time.[45] I must use the word "appear" because this study was not designed to produce conclusive evidence, as all men were given pomegranate juice: the only way to prove a protective effect would be via a randomised trial, in which men are randomly assigned to either a group taking the food supplement or to a an untreated group (ideally receiving a placebo), and evidence of benefit can only come from comparing the outcomes in these two groups.

There have been a few such randomised trials and Hackshaw-McGeagh in 2015 published a systematic review article of these studies aimed at assessing whether dietary/nutritional interventions can slow down cancer progression and mortality. The key findings were as follows:[46]

- One of the studies of lycopene supplements showed benefits.

61

- One of the genistein (soy) trials showed benefits, though some bias was found in the study design.
- Another study found benefits for both soy or soy plus linseed (but again thought to have a risk of bias).
- A well-conducted study found that Pomi-T (a tablet containing broccoli, turmeric, pomegranate powders plus green tea extract) significantly reduced the rise in PSA.
- Another randomised trial also showed a reduced rise in PSA with a different supplement (tablets with soy, isoflavones, lycopene, silymarin and antioxidants).

It has been argued that studies showing a reduction in PSA rise do not really prove that the used supplement is beneficial, as more relevant end points would be tumour size reduction or mortality. There has been, however, an update of the Pomi-T study in which imaging was used and PSA changes were seen to correlate with MRI tumour progression; this follow-up study also showed that tumour improvement in the MRI was seen only in eight men who had taken Pomi-T.[47] The authors of the systematic review article[46] argue that larger, well-designed trials are required to prove beyond doubt the benefits of these dietary supplements; the reality, though, is that any such trials are unlikely to be done. Large expensive trials usually take place when financed by the pharmaceutical industry, but they only finance studies of new medications that will be covered by a patent thus guaranteeing subsequent profits. It is very difficult to get financial support for large studies of food supplements, which are not protected by a patent.

Vitamin D

Vitamin D deficiency in humans is primarily associated with bone disease, though there is increased evidence of an association between vitamin D deficiency and various age-related chronic diseases including Alzheimer's, Parkinson's, cognitive impairment and cancer risk, particularly for colorectal cancer but possibly prostate cancer as well. Vitamin D can be acquired from some foods but is mostly produced by our skin when exposed to the sun: vitamin D deficiency is more common at higher latitudes, where there is more limited exposure to the sun particularly in the autumn and winter months, and in the black population of temperate countries as the skin pigmentation reduces vitamin D production. The association between vitamin D deficiency and prostate cancer has been assessed or discussed in many medical articles, sometimes with conflicting results or conclusions. Schwartz in a recent commentary concludes that there is good evidence of an association between vitamin D deficiency and increased risk of high-grade more aggressive, rather than the low-grade, prostate cancers.[48] More recently Nyame reported an association between low vitamin D levels and more aggressive prostate cancer and commented on previous studies suggesting that vitamin D supplementation may slow down the PSA increase.[49]

A report published in 2016 showed that vitamin D supplementation slows aging in the nematode worm Caenorhabditis elegans:[50] this was reported by the media as vitamin D possibly holding the key to longer life. I think it will be worthwhile watching this space and see what further data might come out regarding the vitamin D link to various conditions, and not just prostate cancer. In the UK, Public Health England (an agency of the Department of Health) issued a recommendation on 21 July 2016 for all adults to take a daily supplement containing 10 micrograms of vitamin D either just in autumn and winter (if there is reasonable exposure to the sun in spring and summer) or throughout the year for those with little skin exposure (care home residents) or with dark skin (Africans, Afro-Caribbeans, South Asians) that may prevent adequate vitamin D production in the skin even during the summer.[51] As some studies (but not all) found an increased risk of prostate cancer with high levels of vitamin D, as well as low levels, it seems prudent not to overdo the vitamin D supplementation and stick to the recommended daily dose (10 micrograms in the UK, equivalent to 400 International Units).

What are my own personal conclusions on diet and food supplements?

- Dietary advice on preventing prostate cancer focuses on increasing consumption of various vegetables, legumes, fruits, nuts, fish and sea foods and limiting (but not eliminating) consumption of dairy products, red meat, eggs: the evidence of benefit for prostate cancer prevention is limited, but this diet is also an excellent diet to reduce the risk of other cancers and cardiovascular disease.

- Some studies suggest that poultry is protective but eating poultry skin might increase the risk of prostate cancer.
- Processed red meats have been classified as carcinogens by the WHO. Do we need to eat them at all?
- There is an opinion in the literature that while many foods could possibly be beneficial, the effect of individual foods might be enhanced when taken together (synergistic effect). As in real life it is difficult to eat all or most of the good foods on a daily basis, the use of supplements like Pomi-T (with extracts of four potentially beneficial foods) is tempting. There is some evidence that Pomi-T might slow down progression of prostate cancer even after diagnosis.
- Vitamin D supplements seem desirable: do not exceed the recommended daily dose (In the UK 10 micrograms = 400 International Units) as the relationship with prostate cancer in some studies was U-shaped (increased risk both with inadequate and with excessive intake).
- Beware of some supplements: selenium and vitamin E were thought to protect against prostate cancers but studies with high-dose supplements have shown adverse effects. Thus, enhance vitamin E intake via consumption of appropriate amounts of known source foods, rather than supplements.

Exercise

If we could give every individual the right amount of nourishment and _exercise,_ *not too little and not too much, we would have found the safest way to health.* (Hippocrates, 5th century Before Christ). Exercise is known to be very important to achieve good health, but what is the impact of exercise in men with prostate cancer?

- Physical inactivity and obesity are thought to be risk factors for prostate cancer: though one study suggested exercise decreased the risk of prostate cancer in white American men but not black men.[52] It is plausible that exercise might be beneficial even after the diagnosis. For instance one study suggested that exercise (walking briskly for three hours per week or more) might reduce the risk of prostate cancer progression[53] and a review article pointed towards survival benefits from exercise with various cancers including prostate.[54] There is also some experimental work that provides support for the hypothesis that exercise might improve prostate cancer outcomes.[55, 56] As often is the case with many medical topics, the evidence is not absolutely definitive, but seems to point in the direction of exercise giving benefits to prostate cancer patients.

- We need to be physically fit to undertake prostate cancer treatment, particularly surgical treatment.
- Most of the studies on exercise in prostate cancer patients have been conducted in patients on androgen-deprivation therapy and they suggest that exercise could (in part) counteract some of the side-effects of treatment. A range of benefits have been demonstrated, mostly enhancement of the quality of life, improved physical and mental health and cardiorespiratory fitness, but possibly also some benefit in reducing the body mass index, preserving sexual activity (see for instance the article by Cormie and others)[57] and possibly a reduction of the treatment-induced osteoporosis.[58] Most of the studies were small and over a short period of time, and were unsuitable to look at whether there could be more substantial benefits such as a reduction in mortality.
- Exercise is good for depression in general and specifically in cancer survivors: more exercise gives a better response.[59]
- Exercise, including pelvic floor exercises, is beneficial at counteracting some of the side-effects of prostatectomy: not just urinary incontinence[60] but erectile dysfunction as well.[61]

How much exercise? I have seen this recommendation in a document that you can download from the Prostate Cancer Foundation website:[43] *Exercise as much as you are able and aim for a vigorous intensity.*

If you walk for exercise, walk as briskly as you can (three plus miles per hour), and try to add bouts of jogging. Vigorous exercise requires close to maximal effort in which your heart beats rapidly and you are sweating. Such activity includes running, vigorous swimming, or fast bicycling. Aim for vigorous exercise for 30 minutes on most days if you are able.

David Tomas, in his book, recalls how he suffered so many side-effects of androgen-deprivation therapy, but then he realised the dream of his life: buying and living in a canal narrowboat. And with the narrowboat journeys came a change of focus but also plenty of fresh air and exercise: he started feeling better.[6]

If men with prostate cancer ask the question of how they can help themselves, exercise alongside diet and fighting spirit are the obvious answers. Football might be a particularly beneficial exercise activity as it may also promote social support,[62] though in practical terms it might be more difficult to organise.

Fighting spirit

If you have been told you have cancer, you have to "fight" it. Don't you? The fighting cancer spirit is epitomised by the cover of a book written by Annette and Richard Bloch[23] (see Figure 4) and is well reflected in the popular health literature.

The essence of the "fighting cancer" message is that cancer treatment is not "their" battle (a battle decided and conducted by the doctors, and other healthcare workers, who treat us), it is "our" battle.

If you do a search of Amazon books with the term "fighting cancer" you will find a lot of books! The topics covered by these books fall into these categories:

- Cancer fighting foods and diets.
- Using "natural remedies" or vitamins or antioxidants.

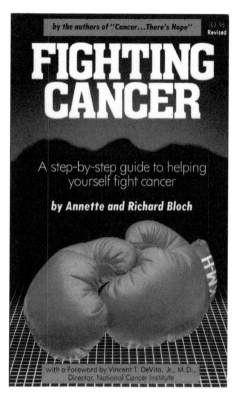

Figure 4. The front cover of this book emphasises the importance of the fighting cancer spirit.

- Fighting depression and developing a "fighting spirit" (or "positive thinking") to achieve good outcomes as opposed to "helplessness/hopelessness" leading to poor outcomes.
- Fighting cancer from within (use the power of your mind for healing and, perhaps, to boost the immune system).
- Mental coping strategies and psychological support.

So, is there any merit in these strategies? Let us look at each of these strategies.

Food and diets

In my opinion, there may be some merit in this (see diet section in this book).

Natural remedies, vitamins, antioxidants

Again, there might be some merit in this strategy, but you also need to be careful. The evidence of benefit sometimes is weak and, more importantly, sometimes there may be risks if you take supplements at high doses. Check from more than one source (and from authoritative sources) before you start taking anything. Vitamins (with the exception possibly of vitamin D in countries with limited exposure to sunlight) and antioxidants are usually best taken via a good diet rather than supplements. You also need to be aware that for some of these products the response curve might be U-shaped: in other words, there may be benefits from some supplements at low doses (particularly if your blood levels were abnormally low) but higher doses might actually be detrimental and bring about worse outcomes. A good example of this might be Vitamin E (see chapter 20 of this reference book).[3]

"Fighting spirit" and "fighting cancer from within"

This is very complex topic, to which I cannot properly do justice. There are lots of publications on this and I only had a quick look at some of them. I am not a specialist in this field either. Nevertheless, I will offer my "take" on this: these are tentative conclusions based on limited knowledge and limited reading.

In November 2002 Mark Petticrew and colleagues published a review article that reviewed 26 previous studies: some of the studies showed an association between fighting spirit or absence of helplessness/hopelessness and either longer survival or lower cancer recurrence, but others did not.[63] The authors concluded that: *good evidence in this subject is still scarce... there is at present little scientific basis for the popular lay and clinic belief that psychological coping styles have an important influence.*[63] I have not mastered the details of these 26 studies but, when the majority of the studies do not show a benefit, there can be at least three possible explanations:

a) Positive thinking and absence of helplessness/hopelessness have no influence on outcomes (as suggested by the authors of this study).

b) Positive thinking and absence of helplessness/hopelessness have some influence on outcomes but not the two outcomes assessed in this review (survival and cancer recurrence).

c) Positive thinking and absence of helplessness/hopelessness have some influence on these outcomes but only in specific circumstances, say only with some cancers or in certain specific circumstances, say early treatment (when there is still a chance of cure) as opposed to late palliative treatment.

When the above study was published, a commentary appeared in the same medical journal.[64] The commentary noticed that there is a myriad of patient support websites for cancer patients, all extolling the need to be positive, whereas cancer websites for doctors tend to concentrate on treatment modalities, rather than coping strategies. The commentary then concluded that perhaps the systematic review had looked at the wrong outcomes: having a fighting spirit might have little impact on outcomes like survival and relapses, but may have something to do with the ability to cope better.

Some of the more recent articles also point towards positive thinking improving the quality of life or reducing distress. One study, based on breast cancer survivors' recollection of their illness, reported that psychological distress was perceived as the worst experience, even more frequently than either chemotherapy or the cancer diagnosis.[65] In the same study breast cancer survivors identified fighting spirit as the main piece of advice they would give to newly diagnosed breast cancer patients.[65]

One particular recent study, that looked at the psychological response in the period one to three months after the breast cancer diagnosis, did demonstrate correlation between the absence of helplessness/hopelessness and longer disease free survival.[66] And in another study pessimism among prostate cancer survivors (not believing that most cancers can be cured) was associated with increased mortality.[67]

The issue of the impact of positive thinking earlier in the treatment course (when the ability to cope might translate in a better ability to choose or complete treatment) as opposed to the terminal illness phase (when a patient may consider it a relief not to be involved in a seemingly never-ending fight and might be looking forward to a good death) is something that appears in some of the published studies, and it makes sense to me. For instance, having a fighting spirit has been associated with less distress amongst newly diagnosed breast cancer patients, but not amongst the long-term cancer survivors.[68] Similar conclusions were reached in another review article: fighting spirit in the early stage was associated with better adjustment, whereas its usefulness in advanced cancer was found to be contentious.[69]

While some believe that positive thinking or fighting spirit bring about better outcomes via a boost to the immune system, I have not seen any evidence myself that this is how it works. Nevertheless, there seem to be genuine benefits from these mental attitudes.

Finally, can I refer to one of Joan Baez's song on this? *We shall overcome.* If I take on a challenge, I like to listen to this song. I know these words were said in a completely different context, but the "fighting spirit" principle still applies. With determination, we can all achieve better outcomes and better quality of life and, sometimes, even a longer life.

Or shall I quote Groucho Marx? *I intend to live forever, or die trying.*

Psychological support

There are some published studies on the potential mental health benefits of psychological support to patients with various types of cancer.[70, 71]

One particular study has looked at the impact of the modalities of the pre-surgical consultation between female breast cancer patients and their surgeon: it was found that being able to assert treatment preferences increased the fighting spirit and decreased anxious preoccupation; the ability of attending companions to ask more questions also reduced anxious preoccupation.[72]

Daniel Carlson in his prostate cancer survivor book reports how important it was, while he was attending for radiotherapy, to be welcomed with a warm greeting and smile by all the staff: from the receptionist to the radiation technologist.[7]

Sense of humour

Having a sense of humour helps in many different situations. We all cry at times, especially after the diagnosis or in other distressing situations. You cannot cry all the time, sometimes you need to have a laugh and use your sense of humour.

The thing I liked most in Daniel Carlson book was the title: *Dear Prostate... I thought you were my friend.*[7] The need to use humour as a coping strategy resonates through this book.

The value of humour in health-care settings, including cancer care settings, is recognised in the medical literature.[73]

Strategic approach and setting targets

Cancer, including prostate cancer, is a challenge. You need to make up your mind on how you are going to tackle it. Yes, others will tell you what the treatment options are, but the choice ultimately is yours. And it is up to you to find a coping strategy. To some extent how you respond to the diagnosis of prostate cancer depends on your personality, but how you respond (depression, denial, passive approach or active involvement, fighting spirit) may affect your outcomes. It is also important to see how the prostate cancer fits with your life plans and whether those plans need to change.

Daniel Carlson reports in his book that: *I made up my mind to be as informed as possible as we decided how to proceed.*[7] Alan Lawrenson also took a very proactive approach.[8] David Thomas recalls in his book how depressed he was about his diagnosis of advanced prostate cancer, but then: *I made a decision. I simply wasn't going to sit in a corner and feel sorry for myself. That was not an option. I wasn't going to weep buckets or say "why me" or any of those other things you hear that people do. I decided I'd be as proactive as I could, take an active part in my treatment and live what life I had left to the full.*[6] So, he started reading and researching about his condition, asking questions whenever he attended an outpatient appointment. His inquisitive approach lead him to discover that, on one occasion, the heavy side-effects of androgen-deprivation therapy were due to the incorrect dosage of a medication, and later on he found out that he was actually a candidate for radiotherapy (initially he had not been given that option). David also decided to reorganise his life. This was an opportunity to prioritise and do the things he had always wanted to do: retire, live in a canal narrowboat, find a new partner.[6]

In conclusion, the diagnosis of prostate cancer may require a coping plan but possibly also a new life plan. We need to be clear about what we still want to do in life and what potential side-effects of treatment we want to minimise, in order to achieve our goals.

My target list goes as follows:
- Quality of life is more important than duration.
- However, I am just 60-year-old and I feel my "mission" has not yet been accomplished;
  - I have two sons aged 25 and 23: I would like to see them more settled in their personal and professional life.
  - I have two elderly aunties for whom I am the next of kin.
  - There are still a few things I would like to do in my life, things I have always postponed because of my busy professional life.
  - And what about my wife? Have we not committed to keep each other company for as long as possible?
- Urinary continence is top goal for a good quality of life.
- Remaining sexually active seems strongly desirable.
- I am a "worker", I like to do things and keep myself busy: even if I retired life would not make sense unless I was able to go to the gym on most days, look after the garden, do repair jobs in the house, keep writing, etc.

- Top priority for my prostate cancer treatment is finding the right balance between attempting cure and minimising side-effects and, in the longer term, avoiding the need for androgen-deprivation therapy (or at least delaying it and/or finding coping strategies).

In my professional experience if you set yourself explicit targets and work with dogged determination towards achieving them, you are more likely to be successful.

Making lists and tables or spreadsheets

Making lists has been one of the few areas of fundamental disagreement between my wife and I. I always make lists, she never makes one. My wife might say: what is the point in making lists if you then forget and leave the list at home? To which I will reply: I do not always forget to bring along my list but, if I do forget, having put things in a list means I am also more likely to remember them anyway. I also find that making lists (and reviewing the to do list everyday) gives me an opportunity to prioritise: I can never really do everything I would like or I have been asked to (neither in my personal nor in my professional life), but I can start from the most important or pressing things. The list also allows me to monitor progress: ticked off items give me satisfaction and a sense of progress.

When it comes to my healthcare, I also tend to do bulleted lists of things I want or have to do. My healthcare checklist included the instructions from the hospital on the many things I have to do before and after the prostatectomy, but also included other things I decided to do on the basis of my independent search for additional fighting strategies (say diet, Pomi-T, vitamin D supplements, keeping in touch with my friends as part of morale boosting etc.). Looking at the prostate cancer literature is an opportunity to extract information about beneficial things that other have found about (scientific articles) or done (prostate cancer survivors books) and those things will go into my bulleted list.

You may regard making lists as an idiosyncrasy but, actually, when it comes to healthcare lists save lives! Gawande was a renowned American surgeon with an interest in patient safety, when he was approached, in 2006, by the World Health Organisation (WHO) with the aim of developing a global programme to reduce avoidable deaths and harm from surgery. We all occasionally hear about surgical disasters in the media, such as patients having the wrong (healthy) kidney being taken out instead of the diseased one, or having been given a medication to which they were known to be allergic. The idea behind Gawande's checklist was that errors usually arise from not making proper use of what we know as opposed to having inadequate knowledge. The story behind the checklist is in one of Gawande's books.[74] Out of this concept came a 19-item checklist sponsored by the WHO and intended for global use: the list is not just about checking a few factual bits of information but also about building the team spirit (confirm that all team members have been introduced by name and role) and listing or anticipating what critical events might take place (say severe blood loss). When the WHO checklist was implemented in eight hospitals across the world, it led to a surgical mortality reduction from 1.5% to 0.8% and to a reduction of other complications from 11% to 7%.[75]

Tables and spreadsheets then. If you have to read a lot of medical articles, there is a real risk of getting lost in the detail: normally all I do is to read the abstract and look at the tables; I will go in the detail of the long text only if I need to clarify a particular point. So, suppose you have read Dr Chodak's book[2] with the aim of making up your mind on how you would like your prostate cancer to be treated and as the basis for a discussion with your specialist: well, there are 42 chapters and 436 pages in this book. You may have highlighted the key bits of information or taken notes, but there is a real risk of getting lost in the detail, at which stage you might turn to your specialist and say "just do what you think is best". Alternatively, you could just look at the key tables in the book. Suppose you are thought to have a localised prostate cancer, in the end focus on Tables 16.2 and 17.1, all the key bits of info are there. Which side-effects are you most worried about and you would rather avoid? Do you seem to be an optimal patient for your preferred treatment modality? You can make a list of questions to ask your specialist doctor(s) based on those tables and other parts of the book. However, to start with, you need to know precisely what is your condition: Jay Cohen in his book (page 132)[5] urges you to do a table (or spreadsheet) with all your key facts (PSA, biopsy Gleason score, presumed cancer stage, risk level, etc.), you cannot look at the range of possible treatment strategies without knowing the basic facts. We are all facing difficult decisions in either our personal or professional life: typically, there are lots of data there, lots of facts and contradictory bits of information. Bulleted lists (of facts, of pros and cons) and spreadsheets or tables are a key strategy to capture and summarise the key facts. In my experience if you look at the data reorganised in a tidy and logical way, the data will talk back to you and suggest what seems to be the best option and the possible way forward.

The importance of your partner

It has been known for some time that having a partner confers a small but real survival advantage. This may apply to both men and women, but possibly more to men than women. Back in 1977 the American cardiologist James Lynch wrote a book arguing that death from heart disease was more common among people who lived alone or had never been married.[76] A more recent article from the USA has confirmed that the death rate for the unmarried (widowed, separated/divorced, never married) is higher than for the married (highest risk is for the never married) and the introduction in this article refers to other studies in different countries with similar findings.[77] Another review study, pooling data from 53 separate studies, showed that marriage decreased the mortality risk by about 6%.[78] Interestingly a subsequent Italian study looked at both cohabitation status, as well as marriage, and showed that both reduced mortality: and in this study it was men more than women who experienced reduced mortality when married or in cohabitation.[79]

It is likely that the small survival advantage, from having a partner, might also apply to individuals with cancer. A study of patients with haematological malignancies undergoing stem cell transplant has showed that patients in a relationship (married or living together) had a longer survival than single patients.[80] It was suggested in this article that patients in a relationship might benefit from both practical and emotional support; a trend towards stronger fighting spirit was also noticed in patients in a relationship. There are also some studies specifically for prostate cancer suggesting a lower mortality in married men such as the one by Tyson and others.[81]

But what can you do if you are single man with no intention, inclination or interest in changing your status? Well a number of studies have looked at mortality risk (not specifically prostate cancer mortality) and found that it is not just about being married or cohabiting, what also might matter is the strength of your social network: having children or other close relatives, having friends, the frequency of contact with relatives and friends. If you are single you may want to consider the benefits of other sources of support and social interactions, including prostate cancer support groups.

Finally, you may happen to be single but with an aspiration to find a partner, and you might think that because of your age and your prostate cancer diagnosis you are not really likely to find a new partner. If this is what you feel, may I suggest that you read the book written by David Thomas?[6] I found this book very inspirational. David was 53 years old when he was unexpectedly diagnosed with advanced prostate cancer: the prognosis seemed to be very poor but he responded to androgen-deprivation therapy, though at the price of many unpleasant side-effects. The initial emotional impact of the diagnosis was massive: David had sleepless nights and felt he could not tell anybody (David was separated and not living with his children). But eventually David realised that talking to relatives and to friends was a really important coping strategy. Then David realised that he also wanted to have a new partner: but how difficult this would be for a man with ongoing prostate cancer battling with the side-effects of the medications? I think David had a real stroke of genius: he wrote a profile for a dating website pretending to be his cat describing himself, this was an incredibly original, funny and tender way to do it. I am not surprised at all that soon after David was contacted by a woman, who then became his partner. This book really has to be read, there is a lot to be learnt.

The importance of friends and social support

Apart from your partner (if you have one) and other close relatives, the other most important source of support is friends, colleagues and your social network. At some stage, we need to tell them and most of us like receiving words of sympathy, receiving get well cards or phone calls or visits whilst recovering. And if we tell our friends, we may soon discover that a few others have been diagnosed with prostate cancer, or other cancers: we are not alone, and if they made it we can make it.

If you think it is difficult to tell others about your diagnosis, please read the book written by David Thomas: telling others was the turning point that lifted him from the initial demoralisation and depression.[6] A friend of mine also told me he felt better when he could tell colleagues at work that he had prostate cancer and was awaiting a prostatectomy, as it meant that they could then understand him and his worried behaviour.

Daniel Carlson, a prostate cancer patient who chose radiotherapy, subsequently wrote in his book about the group of cancer patients with whom he sat and talked to everyday, during his 40-day course of treatment: he saw them as fellow-travellers and as a source of good-natured humour that relieved the tension.[7] Mr Carlson also saw this group as a support group: if he was suffering from a particular radiation side-effect, apart from discussing with his radiation oncologist, he also found it quite useful and reassuring when he found out that others had had the same experience at that point in the treatment. This is how he described the interactions with other patients: *Over the forty days of my treatment, fellows would graduate from our little band and new guys would join in their stead. And while the assortment of faces in the room would change, the dynamic would remain the same... It is important to recognise that this sort of group interaction or solidarity may not be appealing to everyone... I met several other patients who, while cordial, were clearly not interested in the sort of convivial dialogue I have described.*[7]

There are a few studies in medical journals that suggest that the extent of the social support or network in patients with cancer (not specifically prostate cancer) is a predictor of lower mortality. For instance Pinquart and Duberstein conducted a meta-analysis (which is a way of combing the results from all the previous appropriate studies in cancer patients) and they reported that a high level of perceived social support reduced mortality by 25%, having a larger social network gave a 20% reduction, whereas being married gave a smaller 12% reduction.[82] Beasley and others reported that engagement in activities outside the home (contacts with family and friends, attendance at religious services, participation in community activities) was associated with lower overall mortality after breast cancer diagnosis.[83] Rottenberg and others also found that having diverse social networks before a cancer diagnosis was associated with better survival in older individuals.[84]

Possible explanations for the influence of social support or network on mortality include:[82]

- Biological: for instance, social support may limit stress-related endocrine changes that may facilitate tumour proliferation.
- Social support influencing health behaviour: for instance, social contacts might prompt to seek a diagnosis or addressing complications earlier.
- Social support facilitating access to healthcare.
- Social support motivating patients to seek more active cancer treatment.
- Psychological: social support may reduce depression, which is known to have influence on mortality.

Apart from possibly reducing mortality, the level of social support may also have other benefits: it has been associated with quality of life in breast cancer survivors,[85] with acceptance and positivity in cancer patients referred for palliative care[86] and with less helplessness/hopelessness and less anxious preoccupation in another group of long-term cancer survivors.[87] For prostate cancer patients, particularly those whose treatment is ongoing, attending prostate cancer patients support group meetings might be a way of strengthening social support.

Prostate cancer support groups

Many hospitals offering prostate cancer treatment have prostate cancer support groups. Alternatively, prostate cancer support groups might be available via your own relevant national prostate cancer charities (in the UK local support groups can be found via the website of *Prostate Cancer UK*, in the USA or Australia you can find support groups via the *Us Too* or *Malecare* websites).

The groups are attended by men with a recent or past prostate cancer diagnosis and they offer a really important opportunity to gain information and, perhaps, a sense of camaraderie. Where have others gone for diagnosis of treatment? What is their experience with a particular surgeon? Have they suffered from similar side-effects and did they find a way to cope or mitigate? It can be really useful to talk to other men who have gone through similar experiences and it can help to reduce fear and anxiety. Some of us may find it difficult to talk about problems "down there" and about feelings and worries, though in my experience it is often helpful and beneficiary (in all sorts of situations) if you can steer yourself to be more open. But I also know of men with prostate cancer who do not want to go to support groups because they just want to forget their diagnosis. They had their surgery as soon as possible to get it out, and now they want to move on. Yes, they know they need PSA checks and that further treatment might be required in future, but the less they think about it the better. We all have our own coping strategies.

Jay Cohen's experience, as reported in his book, is somewhat different.[5] The official support group was not meeting when he was facing the choice of a treatment modality: he ended up in an independent support group, and quite a unique group as well. They were a group of men quite determined to research their condition and seek out any new relevant published studies. It was this group of men who explained him for the first time how a high PSA could also be due to a prostate infection and not necessarily tumour progression. It was this group of men who pointed that new MRI imaging could help better to understand the stage and whether surgery is really indicated. In the end, it was through this group of men that Jay Cohen realised that active surveillance was possible, and it was his preferred option. According to Ralph Blum, the downside of groups without a professional or experienced moderator is that it might be difficult to discuss intimate things such as erectile dysfunction or incontinence.[4]

Prostate cancer is often a chronic disease: some men are on long term androgen-deprivation treatment, others try surgery or radiotherapy with the aim of achieving a permanent cure, but the PSA might start rising again heralding a possible relapse. So, if you made friends in a prostate support group, it is worthwhile to keep going. Jay Cohen says: *we keep meeting because we enjoy it, we like helping newly diagnosed men and each other, we're always coming across new science to discuss.*[5]

Us Too also gives the option to join a Prostate Cancer Online Community: use the link in the Inspire website (https://www.inspire.com/) to join in and log on. Inspire manages discussion groups for various conditions and, on joining, you must indicate you have prostate cancer. Inspire has a set of community guidelines, that we must respect, one of which is a fundamental rule for any support group: *Do not use Inspire as a substitute for, or to give, medical advice.* In essence support groups are an ideal opportunity to compare notes and get opinions, but anything has to be taken with a pinch of salt, and what might have worked for a support group member may not be applicable in different circumstances. We can bring ideas from the support group to our treating physician, but we cannot substitute our treating doctor with a support website. Similarly, *Prostate Cancer UK* also has an online community, though it seems more tightly moderated.

Social class influence on outcomes

There has always been an association between social class and health: in the past, the association was largely explained by poor nutrition and poor sanitation, with infectious diseases being a major cause of death. In more recent times the association between social class and poor health is frequently explained by differences in unhealthy lifestyles such as smoking, alcohol and diet. Underpinning those lifestyles are differences in income and in education.

Differences in treatment outcomes by social class have been reported for almost every condition, thus it is not surprising that they have been reported for prostate cancer as well, even in settings of universal free healthcare where difference in outcomes cannot be explained by inequalities in access to healthcare.[88, 89, 90]

But are the differences in health outcomes in different social classes only due to factors like income and education, which are largely non-modifiable in adult life? A possible important determinant of outcomes is health literacy, which is the ability to obtain, retain and understand information about medical conditions and access to health services. Health literacy is clearly very important for cancer treatment decisions and compliance, and probably largely relates to the patient's educational level. Rayford has commented on the fact that management of prostate cancer patients with low socioeconomic status or low literacy presents a challenge to healthcare professionals.[91]

I am neither an expert in this field, nor a psychologist, but can I put forward my personal interpretation that some of the prostate cancer outcome differences across social classes are, at least in part, due to modifiable behaviours and attitudes? There are behaviours that, although more common in higher social classes, might well be adopted by most and might be conducive to better outcomes, and the list of these individual behaviours include:

- Valuing prevention and trying to keep up-to-date with evidence regarding healthier lifestyles (through websites, healthy lifestyle magazines or newspaper reports).
- Desire to understand any new diagnosed condition and to find out about treatment options: willingness to seek information online or from books.
- Asking questions at medical consultations and requesting a second opinion.
- Investigating how best to make use of the healthcare facilities.
- Seeking any possible additional health-enhancing strategies (such as diet, exercise, complementary therapies, fighting spirit).

- Recognising the importance of (and seeking) the support from relatives, friends and support groups.
- Recognising the importance of adhering to any healthcare instructions received (say for pre- or post-surgical care) but also the need to report promptly side-effects or to seek new consultations if response is poor.
- Having a can-do attitude.

The above bulleted points reflect my personal and professional experience, buy I notice Ann Bell has reached similar conclusions when comparing how women in high or low socioeconomic status seek health information.[92]

Sex life

Whatever your age, if you are sexually active when you are diagnosed with prostate cancer, you probably want to continue to be so. A number of studies has shown that quite a proportion of both men and women are sexually active later in life and this proportion has increased over the past decades, probably as a result of the availability of medications to treat erectile dysfunction. This shift in sexual activity age boundaries, and a general increase in age and longevity, mean that some would now say "60 is the new 40". An association between sexual activity and good health in older men and women has been described in a number of studies, though this raises the issue of what is the cause and what is the effect. It is possible that the relationship is bidirectional: good health may encourage sexual activity, but sexual activity may also contribute to good health.

Prostate cancer treatment can have an impact on the ability to have intercourse. The option with the least impact is active surveillance, and this is probably the best option anyway, when appropriate. However Xu, in his survey of American men diagnosed with prostate cancer, reported that many were driven to choose immediate surgery by fear and a desire "to take it out" as soon as possible (*I would rather live than have sex*) when actually most of the men in this group had low-risk Gleason 6 cancers that could have been managed with active surveillance.[14] The greatest impact on sex life seems to be from andro-gen-deprivation therapy, which is frequently associated with decreased sex drive and erectile dysfunction (see chapter 14 in Chodak's book).[2] Because of this, and other side effects, as well as the time-limited response achievable with androgen-deprivation therapy, many (especially in the "younger" age group) may prefer prostatectomy or radio-therapy and resort to androgen-deprivation therapy only if the prostate cancer recurs. When facing the choice between prostatec-tomy and either external radiation or brachyherapy, Table 16.2 in Chodak's book summarises the key differences:[2] erectile dysfunction problems seem to be more common with prostatectomy, though nerve-sparing can make some difference. The timing of any side-effects also seems to be different: prostatectomy has an immediate impact followed by some recovery of both continence and erectile function, whereas with external radiotherapy the side-effects may occur even years later and some will experience anejaculation (Chodak's book chapters 16 and 18).[2]

For those undergoing a prostatectomy the key issues in relation to sexual activity are:

- Penile rehabilitation helps (see relevant section in this book).
- You need a period of recovery: it can take up to two years to recover.[93]
- Erectile dysfunction medications can improve the proportion of men who can have sex.[94]
- The proportion of men having good erectile function recovery post-prostatectomy is extremely variable in different studies: younger men and those with bilateral nerve sparing have better outcomes. Mulhall in a review article has reported this frequency as follows:[95]
    - Bilateral nerve sparing: on average 50% of men recovered sexual function;
    - Unilateral nerve sparing: on average 34% recovered sexual function.

- Penile shortening: the average shortening is only one centimetre but the length can return to what it was within four years, particularly if the nerve bundles are preserved (Chodak's book chapter 9).[2]
- All men undergoing a prostatectomy will have dry orgasms (anejaculation). Is it much fun having sex with a dry orgasm? Some men report this decreases their pleasure during sexual activity (Chodak's book chapter 9).[2] A survey of men questioned about orgasmic dysfunction after a prostatectomy reported that:[96]
  - 4% had a more intense orgasm;
  - 22% had no change in orgasm intensity;
  - 37% had decreased orgasm intensity;
  - 37% had no orgasm at all.
- Painful orgasm (dysorgasmia): in a survey of men who had undergone prostatectomy, 14% reported pain during the orgasm but with variable frequency. Within the 14% reporting pain:[96]
  - 19% had pain rarely;
  - 35% had pain occasionally;
  - 13% had pain frequently;
  - 33% had pain always.
- Poor sexual function arising from depression.
- Though most studies focus on the men's sexual function, one study reported that the female partners' sexual function was also adversely affected by the prostatectomy; some couples reported that when penetration was not achieved, sexual satisfaction was pursued through oral or manual stimulation.[97]
- The sexual quality of life of men-who-have-sex-with-men (MSM) is also affected by prostate cancer and there is less MSM-specific survivorship support; as for heterosexual men, the greatest impact seems to be for single MSM men.[98]
- Pelvic floor exercises, though normally undertaken to reduce urinary incontinence, can also improve erectile dysfunction even when started 12 months after the prostatectomy.[61]

- It may be useful to recognise that there are other routes to intimacy. Degauqier and others, in the context of the impact of aging on sexuality, suggest that the most decisive factor: *is the ability to adapt to a more sensory sexuality, less focused on performance and coitus.*[99] Ralph Blum gives a similar account in his book: *Another woman confessed that when her husband lost his libido and his ability to have erections, he closed off emotionally, totally shut her out. "But for me, " she said, "sex is not just about erections. What I want most is emotional closeness, and I need to be touched, cuddled, held. I need my man to find other ways of expressing love and being intimate."*[4]

This is perhaps the most difficult topic to discuss with other men who have had a prostatectomy, it is easier to discuss the incontinence issue. The only man I talked to about this said he was quite happy and capable of having sexual intercourse with the help of sildenafil.

I think this is going to be a significant challenge for many men undergoing a prostatectomy and it may require a multipronged approach. Many surgical units have prostate cancer survivorship nurses, who can help with this, but men need to be able to discuss this with their partner as well as healthcare workers, and they need a willingness to try the many possible different approaches.

Tumour stage and grade

Before the prostatectomy procedure the prostate cancer stage can be estimated on the basis of the clinical assessment and imaging (this is the initial "clinical stage"), whereas the cancer Gleason grade is based on the histopathology (histology) reports of the prostatic biopsies. Chodak in chapters 2 and 3 of his book explains how the tumour stages and grades are scored.[2] The problem is that these stages and grades assigned before the prostatectomy may not be accurate: it is only when the prostate and seminal vesicles are removed during the prostatectomy (sometimes with the regional lymph nodes) that it is then possible to have a final grade (which can be different from the Gleason grade based on the biopsies) and a final stage ("pathological stage").

The information about the tumour stage and grade can be combined with the PSA value to classify all the localised prostate cancers in one of three risk groups: low risk, intermediate risk and high risk (Chodak chapter 5):[2] this classification has prognostic value and helps to identify appropriate treatment options, see Table 4.

Table 4: classification of prostate cancers based on EAU guidelines: this is based on the original D'Amico risk stratification.[17]				
Categories and sub-categories	Localised			Locally advanced
	Low-risk	Intermediate -risk	High-risk	
Definition	PSA < 10 ng/ mL and Gleason score < 7 and Stage T1 or T2a	PSA 10-20 ng/mL or Gleason score 7 or Stage T2b	PSA > 20 ng/ mL or Gleason score > 7 or Stage T2c	Cancer extends outside the prostate capsule (stages T3-T4) and/or into the lymph nodes, but no metastases

It is not always straightforward to apply the risk stratification in the above Table. Take PSA for instance, I believe it is meant to be the last PSA value before surgery, but what if (like myself) you had four PSA tests over less than two months in the run up to my prostatectomy? Well, my PSA results were 21, 15, 17, 16: the mean PSA value was 17 and the median value 16.5, my urologist seemed happy to classify me as "intermediate". Clinical staging was also problematic for me as my MRI showed a small 8mm lesion but in the anterior part of the prostate midline: tumours like this are less common than those in the posterior part of the prostate and affect both sides of the prostate, but not because they are large but rather because of their central position. Thus, as far as the stage is concerned, was I really a T2c (cancer on both sides) that would place me in the High-risk category? My urologist seemed to be happy to classify me as a T2b (cancer in >50% of one side) though on the basis of the size perhaps I could even be a T2a. Others have commented on the fact that subdividing the T2 category does not appear to provide useful prognostic information as it seems unlikely that a small midline tumour (T2c) is worse than a large unilateral tumour (T2a).[100] In the end you need to ask your urologist what they think is your clinical stage and risk category.

Before your prostatic biopsies are taken, you can estimate your probability to have (or not) a prostate cancer on the basis of your age, race, PSA result, family history, digital rectal examination and any previous biopsy results. I used the risk calculator on the University of Texas Health Science Center website at http://deb.uthscsa.edu/URORisk Calc/Pages/results.jsp. My risk report (based on Caucasian race, age 60, PSA 17, no family history of prostate cancer, normal digital rectal examination, no previous biopsies) was as by Figure 5: 61% probability of not having cancer, 23% of a low-grade cancer (I presume they mean Gleason 6) and 16% probability of a "high-grade" cancer (I presume they mean Gleason score 7 or above).

The above calculator did not allow me to enter the positive MRI finding, which probably increases the probability of cancer, but by how much? I do not think this calculator is really designed to take into account any MRI findings, but in my case I do not thing this really mattered a lot, my probability of having a prostate cancer was high enough to justify doing biopsies (as much as I hated the idea).

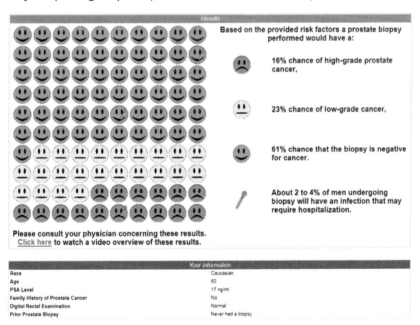

Figure 5. My probability of having prostate cancer detected in the biopsies according to the calculator at http://deb.uthscsa.edu/URORiskCalc/Pages/results.jsp.

A couple of weeks after the prostatic biopsies have been taken, the histology report should be available: in the UK the report will normally be produced in compliance with the guidelines issued by the Royal College of Pathologists.[100] The key findings in the biopsies histopathology (histology) report are:

- Whether cancer is present and, if so, the overall Gleason score that defines the grade.
- The number of biopsy cores taken and how many cores showed cancer on each side.
- The overall percentage of cancer tissue out of all the biopsies.
- Whether there is evidence of extraprostatic extension (cancer outside the prostate capsule): though this is not always easily determined in biopsy specimens.

The biopsy histology results, together with the clinical stage, should allow a meaningful discussion about treatment options. A significant proportion of prostate cancers have a Gleason score of 6 (3+3): Gleason 6 has a benign type of biological behaviour and it would be rare for a Gleason 6 to give extra-prostatic extension or metastases or relapses after prostatectomy. Thus, the title of chapter 5 in this textbook is: *should Gleason score 6 still be called cancer?*[3] Most Gleason 6 cancers may not require immediate treatment, particularly if they meet the other criteria for low-risk as shown in Table 4, and active surveillance, as described by Chodak in chapter 8 of his book, would be adequate.[2] However, there is a big important proviso! Gleason score 6 can be considered definitive and reliable only if based on the assessment of the whole prostate, as it would be done after a prostatectomy. If the Gleason 6 score is based on biopsy results, there is a possibility of "undergrading": in other words the biopsies might have missed the more malignant parts of the cancer, thus the real score might be higher than 6 in about 25% of cases undergoing repeat biopsies, as discussed in chapter 25 of the reference textbook.[3] Over time it is also possible that some grade 6 cancers may progress to higher grades: though the risk of progression seems to be only about 1% per year.[3]

After Gleason grade 6, the next one up, in terms of worsening prognosis, is Gleason 7, but this group is now subdivided into two types: 3+4 (the main tumour is grade 3) and 4+3 (the main tumour is grade 4). The latter (Gleason 7 with 4+3 pattern) is more aggressive. Although active surveillance is usually recommended only when Gleason score is 6 or less, men with Gleason score of 7 (particularly if 3+4 rather than 4+3) have been included in some active surveillance studies (EUA guidelines) in particular circumstances.

If you are considering having a prostatectomy you may want to get an idea of what is the probability of cure (as perhaps prostatectomy is more appealing when the probability of cure is higher) as well as an idea about the probability that your prostate cancer has already spread to the lymph nodes. If the probability of spread to the lymph nodes is high, you may need to have lymph node dissection together with the prostatectomy, or else you might prefer other treatment options. There are a number of ways for doing this such as the Partin Tables or the Kattan Nomogram (Chapter 3 of Chodak's book).[2]

I tried to use the Kattan Nomogram available on the Memorial Sloan Kettering Cancer Center website at https://www.mskcc.org/nomo-grams/prostate/pre-op: the info required is age, PSA, primary Gleason score (the first of the 2 Gleason scores), secondary Gleason score, clinical tumour stage, number of positive biopsy cores and number of negative biopsy cores. I encountered two problems. Firstly, it only allows you to enter a maximum number of 20 negative cores. In my case there had been 11 positive cores and 30 negative cores (I had a lot of biopsies): thus I scaled down my numbers, as what is critical is the percentage of positive cores (I entered 7 positive cores and 20 negative cores). The second problem was the uncertainty about the clinical stage. On the basis of my MRI my urology consultant thought I was probably a T2b, but the histology report on the biopsies stated that on one side there was suspicion (but no certainty) of extra-pros-tatic extension, which could make my stage become a T3a. Thus, I decided to do calculations using the nomograms for both possibilities, the key results are in Table 5.

Table 5. My probability of either not dying from prostate cancer or not having a relapse according to the nomogram at https://www.mskcc.org/nomograms/prostate/pre-op.		
Probability	If I am a T2b stage	If I am a T3a stage
Of not dying from prostate cancer within 15 years	99%	96%
Of not having a prostate cancer relapse with rising PSA within 10 years	59%	55%
Probability of lymph node involvement	3%	4%

My impression was that whether I was a T2b or a T3a possibly it did not make a huge difference, it seemed unlikely I would die of prostate cancer and there was a >50% probability of cure that appeared to justify doing a prostatectomy. At the same time, I may have to accept the fact there is a significant risk of relapse and having to use further treatment modalities such as radiotherapy or androgen-deprivation therapy. The information about the probability of lymph node involvement is important because it helps to decide whether extended lymph node dissection, which carries a higher risk of complications (see chapter 10 in Chodak's book), [2] should be carried out at the time of the prostatectomy. The European Association of Urology recommend that lymph node dissection should be performed when the risk of lymph node involvement exceeds 5%.[17] Using the Kattan Nomogram of the Memorial Sloan Kettering Cancer Center, it seemed that my risk of lymph node involvement was below 5%. However, the European guidelines recommend using a more recent nomogram developed by Briganti and based on a set of patients with a more extensive search for lymph node involvement: it is possible to use the paper version of the nomogram in Figure 1 of the article written by Briganti[22] but it is difficult to get a precise calculation this way. There is an online version of the nomogram at the Knight Cancer Institute website at http://skynet.ohsu.edu/nomograms/prostate/Prostate Nodes.php. Using this calculator my probability of lymph node involvement was 5% (if stage T2) or 16% if I was stage T3.

Another possible explanation for a PSA rise: prostatitis

Initial abnormal PSA: you may not need prostate biopsies if you have prostatitis

If you have done a PSA test, for whatever reasons, and you are then found to have an abnormally elevated result, you are likely to be referred to a urologist who will probably recommend prostatic biopsies. Prostatic biopsies can be unpleasant and give you complications and, especially in the past, tended to trigger a process of overtreatment with many men undergoing aggressive treatment (prostatectomy or radiotherapy) even for non-aggressive cancer types (Gleason 6) that could have been managed with active surveillance. Dr Mark Scholz, a medical oncologist who has co-written a book with Ralph Blum, a prostate cancer survivor, has described this process as follows: *Most men are unaware of the chain of events that will follow if a biopsy reveals the presence of cancer.*[4]

So, if you have been found to have a raised PSA, do you really need prostatic biopsies? Possibly not if any of a number of circumstances that can cause a rise in the PSA did apply to you: Jay Cohen on page 19 of his book gives a list of causes of elevated PSA (other than cancer) and these are reported below.[5]

- Sexual intercourse with orgasm in the previous 48 hours.
- Recent bicycle ride or use of exercise bike resulting in pressure in the prostate area.
- Benign prostate hyperplasia: a generally accepted rule is that the "normal" range increases by 1 ng/ml for each 10cc of prostate. Thus, the upper limit would be 4 ng/ml for a normal 40 cc prostate, but 7 ng/ml for an enlarged prostate measuring 70cc. Dr Scholz recommends that a key strategy to reduce the number of unnecessary biopsies is to measure the prostate size with an ultrasound scan and then correct the reference range value before deciding to do a biopsy (page 83 of his book).[4]
- Prostatitis: of which there are 4 types, see Table 6.

A positive PSA test is an important result that triggers an invasive procedure (prostatic biopsies): any such result should be confirmed on a repeat new sample, the reason being that, sometimes, abnormal results are due to incorrect labelling of the sample tubes (patient's mix-up) or to a laboratory mistake. So, make sure that the repeat blood is not taken the day after sexual intercourse or a long session on an exercise bike. And if you have symptoms suggestive of acute or chronic bacterial prostatitis, you want to be given a course of antibiotics first (four to six weeks of antibiotics with good penetration into the prostate), as they might return the PSA into the normal range. the most effective antibiotics for prostatitis are fluoroquinolones and trimethoprim-sulfamethoxazole.

You need to remember that the PSA test is organ specific (PSA is only produced by the prostate or by disseminated prostate cancer) but not disease-specific: a number of conditions affecting the prostate can result in an abnormal PSA result including prostatitis. Prostatitis is an inflammation of the prostate, often but not always due to infection. It is important to recognise that there are different types of prostatitis. There is a good review article on prostatitis in the Medscape website at http://emedicine.medscape.com/article/785418-overview. I have summarised the key facts in Table 6, but in essence type I and type II are infections and are easier to treat: type III and type IV are largely diagnoses of exclusion (diagnosed after you have excluded infection) for which we do not know well what are the causes or the treatment.

Table 6. Simplified overview of the 4 types of prostatitis as classified by the National Institutes of Health (NIH).

Type	Cause	Symptoms and signs	Treatment
Type I: acute bacterial prostatitis	Bacterial infection	acute onset of – fever, chills, malaise – pain on passing urine, occasionally urinary retention – perineal or rectal pain – Urine culture demonstrates bacterial infection	Antibiotics for 4–6 weeks
Type II: chronic bacterial prostatitis	Bacterial infection	prolonged duration of symptoms – Repeat (relapsing) urinary tract infections arising from bacterial persistence in the prostate – Obstructive symptoms (decreased force of the urinary stream, nocturia) and perineal or rectal pain may be present – Urine culture (can be done after prostatic massage) demonstrates bacterial infection	Antibiotics for 4–6 weeks
Type III: chronic non-bacterial prostatitis, aka chronic pelvic pain syndrome	Unknown	– pain or burning upon urination or during or after sexual intercourse – pain between rectum and testicles – no evidence of infection	Can be difficult to treat: see review article[101]
Type IV: Asymptomatic inflammatory prostatitis	Unknown	– no symptoms: accidental diagnosis when prostatic biopsies are taken and inflammation is showed to be present – no evidence of infection	No satisfactory treatment

All types of prostatitis can result in an elevated PSA but types I and II are usually symptomatic and treated, thus are less likely to be present when prostatic biopsies are taken. Type IV is not associated with symptoms and it probably accounts for the majority of cases in which inflammation is reported to be present in the histology reports of prostatic biopsies. An article by Stancik and others give some good idea of the relative proportion of possible causes of raised PSA resulting in prostatic biopsies: their results are shown in Table 7.[102]

Table 7. Findings in 404 prostatic biopsies as reported by Stancik and others.[102]		
Diagnosis at histology	% of cases	Mean PSA value
Benign prostatic hyperplasia	35.4%	8.2
Prostatitis (presumed type IV)	33.9%	9.3
Prostate cancer	24.8%	11.9
Prostatitis + prostate cancer	5.9%	no data given

In this report, there was no significant difference in PSA levels between prostatitis and prostate cancer. Is there any way to differentiate between these two entities BEFORE we do prostatic biopsies, so that we avoid an unpleasant procedure in patients less likely to have cancer? This is an interesting question and I understand that in some countries, including Italy, it is not uncommon for urologist to recommend a two week course of antibiotics (often with quinolone antibiotics like ciprofloxacin) with the aim of normalising the PSA and avoiding biopsies. The question, of whether antibiotics should be given with the aim of returning the PSA to normal at least in some patients, has been addressed by an article in the Journal of Urology, in which two different authors were asked to make the case either for or against.[103] I would say that on the whole the balance of evidence presented by the two authors is against the routine use of antibiotics, and the key considerations are as follows.

- Men with symptoms suggestive of acute or chronic bacterial prostatitis (types I or II) should be treated with antibiotics (nobody questions this) and the PSA might return to normal (hence no need for biopsies), but this is uncommon.
- In the more common scenario of men having no symptoms, if it was prostatitis it would be type IV, which does not respond to antibiotics.
- Is there a benefit from a three week course of nonsteroidal anti-inflammatory drugs (NSAIDs) to reduce the PSA as reported in reference six of this article? Maybe no harm in trying, but no good evidence that type IV prostatitis responds to NSAIDs.
- There is a potentially significant harm from taking antibiotics (often ciprofloxacin or other quinolone) to try to normalise the

PSA: antibiotics can cause side-effects and often select resistance. Ciprofloxacin is also used for prophylaxis, that is to prevent infection when the prostatic biopsies are taken: if ciprofloxacin has been used before in an attempt to normalise the PSA, there is a high probability of harbouring ciprofloxacin-resistant bacteria at the time of the biopsies and ciprofloxacin prophylaxis may no longer prevent infection after the biopsies.

- PSA frequently fluctuates: thus, the second author of this article recommends that if the PSA is only modestly elevated (say > 4 but <10) it should be repeated after four to six weeks as in a significant proportion of men will have returned to normal (hence no need for biopsies).
- There is also another strategy, though not mentioned in this article: the new MRI modalities may significantly reduce the number of men requiring prostatic biopsies.

Many histopathologists will comment, in their reports, as to whether inflammation is present in prostatic tissue. Thus, I was a bit disappointed when I looked at my prostatic biopsies report and saw no reference as to whether there was inflammation. Particularly when prostate cancer is not detected, mentioning whether inflammation is present or not may help to attempt to address the clinical dilemma of whether the high PSA is caused by a cancer missed by the biopsies or by prostatitis. But even when cancer is present, some patients may wish to go on active surveillance, particularly if a less aggressive Gleason grade 6 cancer is present: however, patients with a PSA > 10 may be told they do not fit the criteria. But what if alongside the cancer there was inflammation as well, could that not contribute to the high PSA? Perhaps active surveillance would be more likely to be considered in those circumstances.

If inflammation is present alongside cancer, would it be beneficial to do something that reduces inflammation? I do not have the answer to this question, but see the discussion below on how inflammation could contribute to the appearance of prostate cancer and how some anti-inflammatory medications might possibly be beneficial.

PSA rise after prostate cancer diagnosis: sometimes it can be due to prostatitis

Patients with prostate cancer and on active surveillance might be prompted to have further biopsies or a curative intervention (prostatectomy or radiotherapy) if their PSA rises significantly. It is important to recognise that patients with benign prostate hyperplasia or prostate cancer are more prone to either urinary tract infections or bacterial prostatitis. Thus, if the PSA rise occurs concurrently with either acute or chronic bacterial prostatitis symptoms, then a course of antibiotics might well be all that is required.

Ralph Blum, in his book, reports how he had his first slightly elevated PSA result in 1990 but he kept refusing surgery or radiotherapy at a time when active surveillance was not yet an accepted protocol, not even for patients like him with a Gleason grade 6 cancer.[4] Unexpectedly, 11 years after his first abnormal PSA, in 2001 there was a sudden PSA rise from 7.4 to 20.3: this was alarming and a curative intervention like radiotherapy was again recommended to him. However, Ralph reported that he was: *feeling lousy – headachy, body aches, running a low fever.* Ralph had no medical background at all but it did occur to him that the elevated PSA could be due to prostatitis (given the associated symptoms) and went to see his family doctor who prescribed a course of ciprofloxacin (an antibiotic with good penetration into prostatic tissue): he got better and his PSA dropped to 9.25, Ralph had bought himself more time on active surveillance![4]

Does prostatitis increase the risk of prostate cancer?

The main issue with prostatitis is that it causes a rise in the PSA, thus resulting in unnecessary biopsies to exclude prostate cancer. However, some researchers have also suggested that prostatitis could actually increase the risk of prostate cancer, though it seems there are conflicting findings in different studies: a good review of the literature dealing with this topic is in chapter 2 of this textbook.[3]

Should we take aspirin or statins?

Interestingly, anti-inflammatory medications such as aspirin or non-steroidal anti-inflammatory drugs (NSAIDs), such as ibuprofen, appear to reduce the risk of prostate cancer, see Chapter 2 in this textbook.[3] How do they do this? Is it because of their ability to reduce inflammation (which might increase the risk of cancer) or through some other mechanism?

And should we take these medications to reduce the cancer risk? Well, it sounds unwise to take NSAIDs just for this reason, because of the risk of side-effects. But what about low-dose aspirin? Aspirin was originally developed and marketed for the treatment of inflammatory disorders at the end of the 19th century. Low dose (for instance 75 mg once daily) can be used to reduce the risk of cardiovascular disease, due to its ability to prevent blood clots, in patients with a previous history of heart attack or stroke; but this has been a controversial issue due to the known increased risk of major bleeding associated with long term use of low dose aspirin. There is now increasing evidence that long-term low dose aspirin use can reduce the risk of various cancers: the evidence seems to be particularly strong for colorectal cancer, for other gastrointestinal cancers and for breast cancer.[104]

In 2016 the US Preventive Services Task Force made clear recommendations for the use of low dose aspirin aimed at reducing both cardiovascular disease and colorectal cancer.[105] The two recommendations in this document are:

- Initiate low-dose aspirin in adults aged 50–59 years who have a 10% risk or greater of cardiovascular disease and a life expectancy of at least 10 years, provided they are not at increased risk of bleeding (check list in Table 8).
- Consider low dose aspirin (but it should be an individual decision) in adults aged 60–69 years who have a 10% risk or greater of cardiovascular disease and a life expectancy of at least 10 years, provided they are not at increased risk of bleeding (again, check list in Table 8).

Table 8. Conditions that increase the bleeding risk and may represent contraindications to the use of aspirin.[105]
• history of gastro-intestinal ulcers;
• history of upper gastro-intestinal pain;
• bleeding disorders;
• renal failure;
• severe liver disease;
• thrombocytopenia (low platelet count);
• use of medications that increase bleeding risk such as anticoagulants or NSAIDs;
• uncontrolled hypertension.

The question, for those already diagnosed with cancer including prostate cancer, is: should we take low-dose aspirin to get a better response to the cancer treatment? This question has been addressed in a recent systematic review article and it was found that, in patients diagnosed with cancer, aspirin reduces mortality; a sub-analysis by cancer type found apparent benefits in colorectal cancer (all-cause mortality reduction 20%), in breast cancer (all-cause mortality reduction 27%) and in prostate cancer (prostate mortality reduction 11%, but all-cause mortality was reduced but not with statistical significance).[106] The authors of this report conclude: *The study highlights the need for randomised trials of aspirin treatment in a variety of cancer … In the meantime it is urged that patients in whom a cancer is diagnosed should be given details of this research, together with its limitations, to enable each to make an informed decision as to whether or not to take low-dose aspirin.*

So, now that I have been diagnosed with prostate cancer, should I go back to my GP to suggest starting low-dose aspirin? It is easy (see below) to establish what is your risk of cardiovascular disease. Currently (age 60, systolic blood pressure 128, very good cholesterol/HDL ratio of 3) my risk of cardiovascular disease over the next 10 years is lowish at 7.8%, I could not justify aspirin just on the basis of this. But if I was 64, even without changes to my systolic blood pressure or cholesterol or weight, my risk would be up to 10.6%. And suppose I was started on ADT and, as a consequence, at the age of 61 my cholesterol/HDL ratio went up to 4.5 and I put up my weight by five kilogrammes: in those circumstances my cardiovascular risk would be up to 10.4%. Well, now that I have been diagnosed with prostate cancer and in the knowledge of my high risk of relapse after the prostatectomy, due to the positive surgical margins, I am inclined to start taking aspirin: maybe it will reduce my risk of prostate cancer relapse as well as my risks of cardiovascular disease and colorectal cancer.

The Prostate Cancer Foundation comments on the possible use of aspirin as follows: *For most men over 60, the balance of risks and benefits favors regular aspirin use. However, the decision to take aspirin regularly should only be made in consultation with a physician, and should consider possible interactions with other medications.*[43] *Substantial data suggest—but do not prove—that regular use of aspirin may lower the risk of lethal prostate cancer. Researchers hypothesize that aspirin inhibits the spread of metastatic cells through its anti-coagulation effects. The evidence is strongest for use before diagnosis, though some studies indicate that post-diagnosis use is associated with a lower risk of disease progression.*[43]

In some observational studies statins, have also been reported to reduce the risk of prostate cancer[107] and of prostate cancer progression.[108] However, not all the studies have showed these beneficial effects, and we need better evidence from randomised trials rather than just observational studies. Statins are a group of lipid-regulating drugs which are taken by individuals with a high risk of cardiovascular disease; they can also cause a range of side-effects including pain or inflammation of the muscles. In the UK the indications for the use of statins, as shown on this website http://www.nhs.uk/Conditions/Cholesterol-lowering-medicines-statins/Pages/Uses.aspx, are:

- Having suffered from any cardiovascular disease (coronary artery disease, angina, heart attack, stroke, transient ischemic attack, peripheral vascular disease).
- More than 10% risk of cardiovascular disease over the next 10 years.

So, what should prostate cancer patients do whilst waiting for better evidence about statins? It sounds as if it is a good thing to take statins only if one meets the criteria for cardiovascular diseases use, but I suspect that a not insignificant proportion of men with prostate cancer might qualify for treatment with statins and may have not been prescribed yet.

How to check what is your risk of cardiovascular disease

The risk can be calculated by your family doctor or else you can use online calculators such as the one at https://qrisk.org/2016/ for UK residents (but ideally you need to know what is your systolic blood pressure and your cholesterol/HDL ratio). USA residents could use the Mayo clinic calculator at http://www.mayoclinic.org/diseases-condi-tions/heart-disease/in-depth/heart-disease-risk/itt-20084942#

Is prostatectomy a cure?

Prostatectomies are often done with the aim of cure, but cure is not a guaranteed outcome. Chodak discusses the chances that the cancer might return in chapter 9 of his book.[2] The most important prognosti-cator seems to be the final Gleason score: sometimes this is different from the Gleason score in the biopsies. Another important prognosti-cator is the presence of "positive surgical margins" which means the cancer extending to the resection margins (thus part of the cancer might have been left behind). However, the extent of the positive sur-gical margins and the location of the positive margins also matter: you can find details of this in chapter 33 of this textbook.[3]

Once you have the histology report on your removed prostate you can make some calculations about your risk of the cancer returning using the Kattan Nomogram available on the Memorial Sloan Kettering Cancer Center website at https://www.mskcc.org/nomograms/pros-tate/post-op. The info required is age, PSA, primary and secondary Gleason scores from the histology of the removed prostate (not the initial biopsies) and other prostatectomy histology report details (sur-gical margins, extracapsular extension, extension to the seminal vesi-cles or not, extension to the lymph nodes or not). If the lymph nodes have not been excised, then the answer is NO to lymph node exten-sion. The key question is how many months one has been without detectable cancer or a rising PSA following the radical prostatectomy: this should be equivalent to the number of months since surgery to the time the PSA rose. So, it seems that whatever the result of the first post-op PSA result is, you need to wait until at least the second post-op test before you have a rising PSA. For those men whose PSA has not risen, the probability of not relapsing increases the longer the PSA remains undetectable. I guess one could use the nomogram to find out the best case scenario (what are my chances if the PSA has not risen after 120 months) or the worst case scenario (what are my chances if the next time I do the test the PSA is rising).

What the nomogram gives us are:

a) The probability of remaining recurrence-free after surgery (this is the probability of not having a biochemical recurrence, defined as the PSA measurement reaching 0.2 ng/mL and confirmed on a repeat measurement).
b) 15-year prostate cancer-specific survival.

I think it is easy to get the nomogram wrong or misinterpret it, so it would be worthwhile discussing it with your urologist. And, as Chodak explains in chapter 19 of his book, a detectable PSA or even a PSA rise does not equate with the appearance of symptoms or metastases, and there would be a range of treatment options.[2] However, I think the key message from this nomogram is clear: you had your prostatectomy, but this is not the time to lower your guard. For most men there is a risk of a relapse, this is our opportunity to further reduce the relapse risk using the strategies discussed in this book (and even if we did not prevent the relapse, we could probably delay it or get physically fitter to face the next challenge). Conversely, even if the risk of relapse is high, there is no point in being unduly pessimistic: relapse is not a certainty and there is something we can do about minimising the risk or attenuating the impact.

After the prostatectomy, the PSA level will be checked at regular intervals: standard PSA tests can detect PSA down to concentrations of 0.1 or 0.2 ng/ml. Although biochemical recurrence is usually defined as a post-prostatectomy PSA more or equal to 0.2 ng/ml on at least two successive tests, some may regard 0.4 ng/ml as a better cut-off value for recurrence. As Dr Chodak explains in chapter 9 of his book there are ultrasensitive PSA tests that can measure PSA at much lower concentrations (0.01 ng/ml or less), but it is not clear whether using the ultrasensitive tests is significantly advantageous.[2] For instance, with the less sensitive tests PSA is undetectable after four to six weeks, but with the tests capable of detecting less than 0.01 ng/ml it may take up to 10 months for the PSA to drop to its lowest post-op concentration (PSA nadir).[2] However, with an ultrasensitive test the PSA nadir (lowest post-op level) is an independent predictor of the risk of biochemical recurrence, and the risk is very low when the PSA is not detected by an ultrasensitive test.[109]

If the risk of recurrence was thought to be high, there is also the option of radiotherapy after prostatectomy (see next section).

Radiotherapy after prostatectomy

There are two scenarios under which radiotherapy might be recommended after a prostatectomy, if there are reasons to believe there is residual cancer left in the prostate fossa (where the prostate was).

ADJUVANT RADIOTHERAPY

This is radiotherapy which is started WITHOUT waiting for evidence of biochemical recurrence (PSA >= 0.2 ng/ml on two consecutive test): it usually takes place within four to six months of the prostatectomy. Adjuvant radiotherapy is offered to patients whose histology report shows at least one of these features:

    i. Extracapsular extension.
   ii. Positive surgical margins.
  iii. Extension to the seminal vesicles.

The case for adjuvant chemotherapy may be stronger when two or even all three features are present. Adjuvant radiotherapy is discussed in page 109 of Dr Chodak's book[2] and in chapter 47 of the reference book.[3] In essence when the above adverse pathological features are present there is an increased risk of biochemical relapse and metastases and the choice is between:

  a) Immediate adjuvant radiotherapy.
  b) Monitoring the PSA and, if the PSA rises, go for either salvage radiotherapy or androgen-deprivation treatment.

With adjuvant radiotherapy, a number of patients, who would not have a biochemical recurrence, are treated unnecessarily and will suffer the side-effects of radiotherapy. With salvage radiotherapy, the number of patients receiving radiotherapy and suffering the side-effects is reduced, but is not clear whether delayed salvage radiotherapy is equally effective as adjuvant radiotherapy. The three studies conducted so far have not given a definitive answer and three more randomised studies are underway.[3] Unfortunately I am now in this situation with my prostate cancer having both extracapsular extension and positive surgical margins: I am more inclined towards salvage (delayed until there is a PSA rise) rather than immediate adjuvant radiotherapy, and my urology consultant seems to be similarly inclined.

SALVAGE RADIOTHERAPY

Salvage radiotherapy is radiotherapy which is undertaken if a patient suffers from a biochemical recurrence after prostatectomy: recurrence is often defined as a PSA level above 0.2 ng/ml, confirmed on a repeat sample.[3] Management of PSA recurrences after prostatectomy is discussed in in chapter 19 of Chodak's book[2] and in chapter 49 of the reference textbook.[3]

A biochemical recurrence is not an immediate threat, at least not for everybody:

- Some men have stable PSA at 0.2-0.4 ng/ml, without further increases.[3]
- Without treatment after five years 37% of men have metastases: the risk of metastases is higher with Gleason 8-10 or when the interval between surgery and biochemical recurrence is shorter or when the doubling time (the time, in months, it takes for the PSA to double) is shorter.[3]
- The median time to metastatic disease is eight years.[3]
- Treatment options include salvage radiotherapy or androgen-deprivation treatment.[3]
- With salvage radiotherapy, it seems that there are better outcomes if initiated at a low PSA, possibly less than 0.33 if Gleason 8–10; with Gleason 7 it does not seem to be critical to start at such a low PSA level.[110]

- With androgen-deprivation, treatment started when PSA is less than 10 ng/ml gives better outcomes in patients with Gleason 7 or greater diseases or with a PSA doubling time of less than or equal to 12 months.[3]

Androgen-deprivation therapy (ADT) after prostatectomy

There are a number of circumstances under which androgen-deprivation therapy (ADT) might be recommended such as early in the disease in combination with radiotherapy, or later in the diseases if metastases have occurred. Patients who relapse after radiotherapy can also be offered ADT, whereas patients relapsing after a prostatectomy might be offered salvage radiotherapy first, and then ADT if they relapse again. One way or another, many men with prostate cancer end up receiving ADT, often on a continuous long-term basis.

ADT involves the use of a number of medications that either lower testosterone (the male sex hormone) or block its effects. Unfortunately these medications can cause many side-effects that affect the quality of life: loss of libido and sexual dysfunction, hot flushes as in post-menopausal women, decreased energy, decline in muscle mass and increase in subcutaneous fat, osteoporosis with increased fracture risk, gynecomastia (increase in the size of male breast tissue), increased risk of diabetes, altered serum lipid levels with possible increased risk of cardiovascular disease, anaemia and tiredness.[3] Chodak discusses ADT in some detail in chapters 23, 25, and 27 of his book.[2] Apart from the unpleasant side-effects, the other main problem with ADT is that it tends to be effective only for a limited period of time, until when there is evolution to what is called androgen-independent prostate-cancer (AIPC) or castration-resistant prostate cancer (CRPC): the two terms are equivalent. After ADT has been started, the time it takes to the prostate cancer to become AIPC seems to be extremely variable: more than a decade in some patients or just a few months in others.

ADT can be regarded as a type of "chemical castration" in the sense that it prevents the testicles from producing testosterone. Surgical castration is rarely used nowadays. Personally, I find the term castration offensive and hurtful, and would prefer the term androgen-independent over castration-resistant.

AIPC used to be really bad news, because it meant the cancer was no longer controlled and patients had or might develop metastases. However, there are now treatment options for AIPC: these are discussed in chapters 30–37 of Chodak's book[2] and in chapters 54, 56 and 57 of the reference book.[3] The problems created by AIPC are discussed also at this Harvard Medical School website: http://www.harvardprostateknowledge.org/androgen-independent-prostate-cancer .

Can our diet have any influence in slowing down progression to AIPC? There is a handful of reports arguing that some of the nutrients and foods that are thought to be good at preventing prostate cancer (resveratrol, lycopene, omega-3 polyunsaturated fatty acid) may perhaps be beneficial in this respect. Although at this stage there is no real hard evidence that diet slows down progression to AIPC, it is worthwhile persevering with a prostate-healthy diet as it is also heart-healthy! One of the side-effects of ADT is increased risk of coronary artery disease: diet and exercise can mitigate this risk. There are a number of studies demonstrating the benefits of exercise, sometimes combined with a diet, in men undergoing ADT: the most commonly demonstrated benefits included loss of fat and better physical functioning. The best study, of those I have seen, included a package of both dietary advice and exercise.[111]

If I will ever need ADT, I will research this treatment modality better. But let me tell you something: as I write this it is two weeks to Christmas and you know what I would like to find under my Christmas tree? A prostate cancer treatment medication strategy that does not rely just on continuous suppression of testosterone, with all the resulting side-effects. Or perhaps Santa has already delivered on this wish, at least in part. For many years we have known about a strategy that reduces the impact of ADT and seems to improve the quality of life: it is called intermittent ADT and consists in alternating ADT cycles with no treatment periods, during which the testosterone recovers. However, not all patients are good candidates for intermittent ADT.

Intermittent ADT is thought to be about as effective as continuous ADT, but better tolerated.[2,3] See also the discussion on the American Cancer Society website at http://www.cancer.org/cancer/prostatecancer/detailedguide/prostate-cancer-treating-hormone-therapy: *in one form of intermittent hormone therapy, treatment is stopped once the PSA drops to a very low level. If the PSA level begins to rise, the drugs are started again. Another form of intermittent therapy uses hormone therapy for fixed periods of time – for example, six months on followed by six months off.* There have been two recent large randomised trials on the use of intermittent ADT and both used PSA monitoring to decide when to restart treatment. The first one was in patients with raised PSA after primary or salvage radiotherapy, but no metastases: the risk of death increased by 2% in the intermittent group, this increase was small and not statistically significant, intermittent treatment gave better quality of life.[112] The second study was in men with metastases: intermittent treatment was associated with a 10% increase in mortality, a bigger difference than in the previous study, though again this difference was not statistically significant; quality of life was better only in the first assessment after 3 months.[113]

Amongst the recent articles in medical journals, the one I found most useful is the one from Lawrence Klotz:[114] a bulleted list of his considered observations and reflections is as follows:

- Unavoidably randomised trials are constrained by protocols, but the best use of intermittent ADT is in individualised approaches that take into account the response to ADT.
- The greatest benefit from intermittent ADT is in patients without metastases, though a smaller subgroup of patients with metastases can also benefit.
- All patients started on ADT who achieve a >95% PSA reduction, to <0.2-0.4 ng/ml after nine months, should be considered for intermittent treatment.
- Then, those patients whose PSA remains <5 ng/ml at six months (after ADT has been discontinued) should be continued on intermittent ADT as they are likely to benefit, the others should return to continuous treatment.

- ADT is restarted when PSA reaches 10–20 ng/ml.
- Quality of life is likely to be better with intermittent ADT only during the intervals not on treatment and only after testosterone has recovered.
- Intermittent ADT is less expensive than continuous ADT!

Klotz concludes his article saying that: *Few treatment approaches offer improved quality of life, reduced comorbidity, decreased cost, and no adverse survival effect... intermittent ADT should be widely embraced.*[114] A similar approach to intermittent ADT is discussed on page 62 of the European Association of Urology guidelines.[17] There have been other studies published since and a systematic review of all the randomised trials, published in December 2015, concluded that: *Intermittent androgen deprivation was not inferior to continuous therapy with respect to the overall survival. Some quality-of-life criteria seemed improved with intermittent therapy. Intermittent androgen deprivation can be considered as an alternative option in patients with recurrent or metastatic prostate cancer.*[115] Surveying the medical literature suggests that not all specialists are enthusiastic about intermittent ADT and, perhaps, the greatest area of uncertainty is whether and when to use in men with metastatic cancer: in a recent article it was suggested that use of intermittent ADT, in a trial of men with metastases, was associated with an increased incidence of ischemic and thrombotic events.[116]

My impression (I might be wrong) is that in some hospitals in my region there is little enthusiasm for intermittent ADT. Liede has recently published the results of an international survey of ADT practices across 19 countries: he showed that there were significant variations in the proportion of patients with non-metastatic prostate cancer receiving intermittent ADT, and the UK with only 10% had one of the smallest proportions.[117] Conversely the proportion of patients on intermittent ADT was 35% in Australia and France, 32% in Canada and Germany, and26% in the USA.[117]

In the past few weeks I also have seen reports in various media about Bipolar Androgen Therapy (BAT): the concept behind this new experimental treatment modality is simple. Androgen deprivation does not work in the long term because of progression to IAPC, due to changes in the androgen receptors, but these changes appear to make the cancer cells more vulnerable to high levels of testosterone. Thus, instead of waiting for testosterone to recover as in intermittent ADT, in BAT treatment there is continuous ADT but with cycles of high-dose testosterone injections; in the only one reported study I have seen some of the men responded well, but it was not a proper randomised trial.[118] We need to wait for the results of the ongoing TRANSFORMER randomised trial in the USA, testing BAT versus enzalutamide in men with metastatic IAPC, and then we will know whether BAT treatment really works.

My take on this complex topic is as follows: medical treatment that does not rely just on continuous suppression of testosterone, with all the resulting side-effects, is a tantalising prospect. For the time being we have intermittent ADT, which may be beneficial but is not appropriate for all patients. Bipolar Androgen Therapy might be another strategy, but we need to wait for the randomised trials results.

Life expectancy

An important consideration when choosing prostate cancer treatment is how long one is expected to live (life expectancy), as shown in Table 17.1 of Dr Chodak's book.[2] Knowing what is one's life expectancy is also important in planning retirement and pension savings: it is a common mistake to underestimate how long one is going to live, and not to make adequate financial provisions. I will use the example of two aunties I have in Italy: they have not made adequate financial provisions, they told me they assumed that, like their parents, they would die in their late 60s or early 70s, they are now aged 90 and 94 years old respectively.

The problem is, you cannot have an accurate estimate, but you can work out a ballpark figure. Table 9 below shows the life expectancy at birth and at age 65 for England (UK) and is based on data from the Office for National Statistics (Life Expectancy at Birth and at Age 65 by Local Areas in England and Wales: 2012 to 2014).

Table 9. Life expectancy in England (UK) according to the Office for National Statistics.		
	Life expectancy in England at birth	Life expectancy in England at the age of 65
men	79.5	83.8
women	83.2	86.2

So, for a man in England at birth the average length of life is 79.5 and some will die before the age of 65, but if a man reaches the age of 65 the average length of life will be 83.8. There are also online calculators, based on the above statistics, which will give the average life expectancy at any age: for instance the calculator at http://www.riskprediction.org.uk/index_lifeexp.php (which applies to the UK population) says that a man in the UK aged 60 has a life expectancy of 82.44 years. This calculator also gives the opportunity of entering some family and personal data for a slightly more accurate estimate. A calculator based on data from the USA is available at https://www.ssa.gov/OACT/population/longevity.html

The problem with all these calculators are:

a) They give the AVERAGE length of life, which by definition means 50% of men will live less and 50% more.
b) Life expectancy is also influenced by lifestyles, social class and whatever medical conditions one may have.

So, the calculators are of limited use. But if you are a man aged 65, when you are diagnosed with prostate cancer, and you are in reasonable good health and live in the UK or the USA (or in others developed countries), you probably do not want to choose a treatment modality recommended for those with a life expectancy of less than 10 years.

A prostate cancer diagnosis is also an opportunity to change your life priorities: work out how much you are likely to live and make a plan for the rest of your life!

Changing the life plans

Some breast cancer survivors have reported that there can be positive aspects to a cancer diagnosis, such as a change in life priorities or having found unexpected support from friends.[65] The title of two studies I have read, cast some light on what particular adaptive strategies might be useful in the long term: see Table 10.

Table 10. Adaptive strategies after a diagnosis of cancer.		
Type of study	Adaptive strategy highlighted in the title	Reference (see bibliography list)
Long term cancer survivors (including prostate) asked to complete a survey 5–6 years post-diagnosis	**Life is precious and I'm making the best of it**: coping strategies of long-term cancer survivors	87
Cancer patients referred to hospice for palliative care (in other words, advanced cancer patients)	**I've had a good life, what's left is a bonus**: Factor analysis of the Mental Adjustment to Cancer Scale in a palliative care population	86

David Tomas' book is a very good example of how a man can change his life plans for the best, after a diagnosis of prostate cancer: he retired, he did what he had always wanted to do (living in a canal narrowboat) and he addressed his loneliness by finding a new partner.[6]

At the moment, my adaptive response is mostly of the type: *life is precious and I'm making the best of it*. I do not know yet whether my cancer will relapse after my prostatectomy, but my relapse risk is high. I may need to undergo radiotherapy at some stage, even if that does not guarantee a cure. Maybe eventually I will be on ADT. Why not to make the best of my life why I am still in relatively good health? Why to carry on delaying all the things I said I would do later in life?

- Why not retire now (age 60) rather than at the age of 65 as I envisaged before this diagnosis? I could take a reduced pension.
- I will carry on living in the UK, but we want to go to Italy more often.
- I always thought I was hopeless at dancing: is this really so? I would like to try dancing classes; it is a good exercise and fun as well (I love watching dancing after all).
- I need to do some more serious gardening: should I try a vegetable allotment?

- I am a reasonable good cook, but I want to expand my repertoire. The choice is between self-learning new recipes or going to some cookery courses.
- I like photography: I could join the local photography club or just take more pictures.
- I need to reorganise and digitalise the family pictures collection (starting from my mother's pictures).
- I always said I would like a go at writing a book.
- Alternatively, I may fancy some Open University courses.
- I intend to carry on going to the gym on most days: but I would like to try a greater variety of fitness classes.
- Most important thing: more quality time with my partner, my family, my friends.

Others may have different priority and aspirations, but a prostate cancer diagnosis may suggest to many that the time has come to start tackling the life aspirations list.

Message for sons and brothers: you are at risk, but you can reduce the risk

So, what should I tell my two sons? One of my worries, the day I was told it really was a prostate cancer, was that this also increases their chances of having a prostate cancer. The increase in risk might be about twofold: see Table 11. The risk is even higher when a brother has prostate cancer or when both the father and a brother are affected.[119] History of breast cancer in a mother or sister also increases the risk, but just slightly.[120] Twice as many chances to get prostate cancer may not sound that bad, but bearing in mind that prostate cancer is the most common cancer in men affecting as many as 14% of us in the UK (lifetime risk, see statistics at http://www.cancerresearchuk.org/health-professional/cancer-statistics/risk/lifetime-risk#heading-One) and 17% in the USA (chapter 12 of reference book)[3], this increase in risk seems to be significant.

Table 11. Risk of prostate cancer on the basis of the family cancer history.		
First degree relatives with prostate cancer	Increase in prostate cancer risk	Reference
Father with prostate cancer	2.35	119
1 brother with prostate cancer	3.14	119
2 or more first degree relatives (father and brother or 2 brothers) with prostate cancer	4.39	119
Mother or sister with breast cancer	1.22	120

The urology consultant who gave me my diagnosis suggested that my sons should start prostate cancer screening (with PSA tests) at the age of 40. Is this what I should tell them? I am a bit wary of telling my sons (currently aged 25 and 23) what to do. They have a mind of their own and, at this age, father's influence is on the wane. The other consideration is that prostate cancer screening is controversial: it has never been recommended in the UK and is no longer recommended in the USA. The argument against prostate cancer screening is that PSA testing inevitably leads to a large number of prostatic biopsies, an unpleasant procedure with occasionally severe complications. Prostatic biopsies may bring about the diagnosis of prostate cancer, which may end up being treated (with surgery or radiotherapy) even in cases when it would have never caused any significant problems. And prostate cancer treatment always has side-effects. In 2012 the US Preventive Task Force recommended that PSA-based screening should no longer be used in the USA, on the basis of an analysis of benefits and harms of screening.[15]

However, having a father with a prostate cancer may tilt the balance in favour of screening. But, what if the knowledge of their father's disease convinced my two sons to undergo early screening and led to them having a prostatectomy in their late 40s or early 50s (with some unavoidable impact on sexual life and perhaps continence), when otherwise they might have had diagnosis and treatment later in life? Conversely, though, waiting for the symptoms to appear later in life might mean requiring more aggressive and more unpleasant treatment, or having to suffer from the progression to bone metastases or even death.

Sons, I cannot tell you precisely what to do. And diagnosis and treatment may change significantly over the next 20 years. But I strongly advise you to:

a) Adopt now a healthy diet and exercise.
b) Keep yourselves well informed.
c) Consider prostate cancer screening, BUT do not start screening without gathering information first: once the screening test has been done, you have started a mechanism in motion that you can no longer stop. You need to know precisely how to respond to a positive PSA result (if that will still be the screening test) and to a subsequent positive biopsy result.
d) Do not panic if you are diagnosed with cancer, you have time to inform yourself and make your choices. Treatment strategies will have changed significantly in 20 years' time, but many of the strategies described in this book, aimed at bringing about better outcomes, will still apply. Be active patients!

Good luck sons, but remember what Seneca the Younger said (1st century AD) about luck: *luck is what happens when _preparation_ meets opportunity.*

BIBLIOGRAPHY

1. Bignardi, G. and others, Cytomegalovirus mononucleosis: risk for fathers of young children. *British Journal of General Practice* 1993; 43:119–120.
2. Chodak, G., *Winning the battle against prostate cancer: get the treatment that's right for you.* Demos Health, 2nd edition 2013.
3. Mydlo, J. H. and Godec, C. J., *Prostate Cancer: Science and Clinical Practice.* Academic Press (an imprint of Elsevier), 2nd edition 2016.
4. Blum, R. H. and Scholz, M., *Invasion of the prostate snatchers: an essential guide to managing prostate cancer for patients and their families.* Other Press, 1st edition 2011.
5. Cohen, J. S., *Prostate cancer breakthroughs: new tests, new treatments, better options – A step-by-step guide to cutting edge diagnostic tests and 12 medically-proven treatments.* Oceansong Publishing, 1st edition 2013.
6. Thomas, D., *They said I had six months to live: surviving prostate cancer – 10 years on.* CreateSpace Independent Publishing Platform, 1st edition 2016.
7. Carlson, D., *Dear prostate... I thought you were my friend: one man's journey through prostate cancer and beyond.* CreateSpace Independent Publishing Platform, 1st edition 2016.
8. Lawrenson, A. G., *An ABC of prostate cancer in 2015: my journey over 4 continents to find the best cure.* CreateSpace Independent Publishing Platform, 1st edition 2015.
9. Kamen, C and others, The association between partner support and psychological distress among prostate cancer survivors in a nationwide study. *Journal of Cancer Survivorship*, 2015; 9:492-9.
10. O'Shaughnessy, P. K., and others, The prostate cancer journey: results of an online survey of men and their partners. *Cancer Nursing*, 2015; 38:E1-E12.

11. Jayadevappa, R. and others, The burden of depression in prostate cancer. *Psycho-Oncology* 2012; 21:1338-45.
12. Prasad, S. M. and others, Effect of depression on diagnosis, treatment, and mortality of men with clinically localized prostate cancer. *Journal of Clinical Oncology*, 2014; 32:2471-8.
13. Nelson, C. and others, The role of spirituality in the relationship between religiosity and depression in prostate cancer patients. *Annals of Behavioral Medicine*, 2009; 38:105-114.
14. Xu, J. and others, Men's perspectives on selecting their prostate cancer treatment. *Journal of the National Medical Association*, 2011; 103:468-478.
15. Moyer, V. A., Screening for Prostate Cancer: U.S. Preventive Services Task Force recommendation statement. *Annals of Internal Medicine*, 2012; 157:120-134.
16. Jacobs, B. L., and others, Use of advanced treatment technologies among men at low risk of dying from prostate cancer. *JAMA*, 2013; 309:2587-2595.
17. Mottet, N. and others, Guidelines on Prostate Cancer. *European Association of Urology*, 2015; 1-137.
18. Feng, T. S., and others, Multiparametric MRI improves accuracy of clinical nomograms for predicting extracapsular extension of prostate cancer. *Urology*, 2015; 86:332-337.
19. Kamrava, M. and others, Multiparametric magnetic resonance imaging for prostate cancer improves Gleason score assessment in favourable risk prostate cancer. *Practical Radiation Oncology* 2015; 5:411-416.
20. Abdollah, F. and others, More extensive pelvic lymph node dissection improves survival in patients with node-positive prostate cancer. *European Urology* 2015; 67:212-219.
21. Harbin, A. C. and Eun, D. D., The role of extended pelvic lymphadenectomy with radical prostatectomy for high-risk prostate cancer. *Urologic Oncology: Seminars and Original Investigations* 2015; 33:208–216.
22. Briganti, A. and others, Updated nomogram predicting lymph node invasion in patients with prostate cancer undergoing extended pelvic lymph node dissection: the essential importance of percentage of positive cores. *European Urology* 2012; 61:480-487.

23. Bloch, A. and Bloch, R., *Fighting cancer: a step-by-step guide to helping yourself fight cancer.* R. A. Bloch Cancer Foundation, 13th edition 2008.

24. Wallis, C. J. D. and others, Second malignancies after radiotherapy for prostate cancer: systematic review and meta-analysis. *British Medical Journal* 2016; 352:i851.

25. Dahl, S. and others, Return to work and sick leave after radical prostatectomy: a prospective clinical study. *Acta Oncologica* 2014; 53:744-751.

26. Hohwü, L. and others, Open retropubic prostatectomy versus robot-assisted laparoscopic prostatectomy: a comparison of length of sick leave. *Scandinavian Journal of Urology and Nephrology* 2009; 43:259-64.

27. Carlsson, S. V. and others, Risk of incisional hernia after minimally invasive and open radical prostatectomy. *Journal of Urology* 2013; 190:1757-1762.

28. Zhu, S. and others. Risk factors and prevention of inguinal hernia after radical prostatectomy: a systematic review and meta-analysis. *Journal of Urology* 2013; 189:884-890.

29. Van Hemelrijck, M. and others. Thromboembolic events following surgery for prostate cancer. *European Urology* 2013; 63:354-363.

30. Secin, F. P., and others. Multi-institutional study of symptomatic deep venous thrombosis and pulmonary embolism in prostate cancer patients undergoing laparoscopic or robot-assisted laparoscopic radical prostatectomy. *European Urology* 2008; 53:134-145.

31. Galvin, D. J. and others. Thromboprophylaxis for radical prostatectomy: a comparative analysis of present practice between the USA, the UK, and Ireland. *Prostate* 2004; 60:338-342.

32. Bannowsky, A. and others, Recovery of erectile function after nerve-sparing radical prostatectomy: improvement with nightly low-dose sildenafil. *BJU International* 2008; 101:1279-1283.

33. Pavlovich, C. P. and others, Nightly vs on-demand sildenafil for penile rehabilitation after minimally invasive nerve-sparing radical prostatectomy: results of a randomized double-blind trial with placebo. *BJU International* 2013; 112:844-851.

34. Köhler, T. S. and others, A pilot study on the early use of the vacuum erection device after radical retropubic prostatectomy. *BJU International* 2007; 100:858-862.
35. Filocamo, M. T. and others, Effectiveness of early pelvic floor rehabilitation treatment for post-prostatectomy incontinence. *European Urology* 2005; 48:734-738.
36. Centemero, A. and others. Preoperative pelvic floor muscle exercise for early continence after radical prostatectomy: a randomised controlled study. *European Urology* 2010; 57:1039-1044.
37. Gould, C. V. and others, Guideline for prevention of catheter-associated urinary tract infections, 2009. *Centers for Disease Control and Prevention* 2009. Can be downloaded from the CDC website: http://www.cdc.gov/hicpac/pdf/CAUTI/CAUTIguideline2009final.pdf
38. Rayman, M. and others. *Healthy eating: the prostate care cookbook.* Kyle Cathie Ltd, 1st edition 2009.
39. Kmietowicz. Z., Processed meats are carcinogenic, says new review of evidence. *British Medical Journal* 2015; 351:h5729.
40. Richman, E. L. and others, Egg, red meat, and poultry intake and risk of lethal prostate cancer in the prostate-specific antigen-era: incidence and survival. *Cancer Prevention Research* 2011; 4:2110-2121.
41. Wu, K. and others, Associations between unprocessed red and processed meat, poultry, seafood and egg intake and the risk of prostate cancer: a pooled analysis of 15 prospective cohort studies. *International Journal of Cancer* 2016; 138:2368-2382.
42. Zhao, J. and others, Is alcohol consumption a risk factor for prostate cancer? A systematic review and meta-analysis. *BMC cancer* 2016; 16:845.
43. *Prostate Cancer Foundation.* Health and Wellness: Living with Prostate Cancer. Diet and lifestyle recommendation. 2015. https://www.pcf.org/wp-content/uploads/2016/10/PCF_HW_Guide.pdf .
44. *Prostate Cancer UK.* Diet and physical activity for men with prostate cancer. June 2015. http://prostatecanceruk.org/prostate-information/our-publications/publications/diet-and-physical-activity-for-men-with-prostate-cancer .

45. Pantuck, A. J. and others, Phase II study of pomegranate juice for men with rising prostate-specific antigen following surgery or radiation for prostate cancer. *Clinical Cancer Research* 2006; 12:4018-4026.

46. Hackshaw-McGeagh, L. E. and others, A systematic review of dietary, nutritional, and physical activity interventions for the prevention of prostate cancer progression and mortality. *Cancer Causes Control* 2015; 26:1521–1550.

47. Thomas, R. and others, Prostate cancer progression defined by MRI correlates with serum PSA in men undergoing lifestyle and nutritional interventions for low risk disease. *Journal of Lifestyle Diseases and Management* 2015; 1:1-8.

48. Schwartz, G. G., Vitamin D in blood and risk of prostate cancer: lessons from the selenium and vitamin E cancer prevention trial and the prostate cancer prevention trial. *Cancer Epidemiology, Biomarkers and Prevention* 2014; 23:1447-1449.

49. Nyame, Y. A. and others, Associations between serum vitamin D and adverse pathology in men undergoing radical prostatectomy. *Journal of Clinical Oncology* 2016; 34:1345-1349.

50. Mark, K. A. and others, Vitamin D promotes protein homeostasis and longevity via the stress response pathway genes skn-1, ire-1, and xbp-1. *Cell Reports* 2016; 17:1227–1237.

51. *Public Health England press release.* PHE publishes new advice on vitamin D. PHE is advising that 10 micrograms of vitamin D are needed daily to help keep healthy bones, teeth and muscles. 21/07/2016. https://www.gov.uk/government/news/phe-publishes-new-advice-on-vitamin-d .

52. Singh, A. A. and others, Association between exercise and primary incidence of prostate cancer: does race matter? *Cancer* 2013; 119:1338-1343.

53. Richman EL and others. Physical activity after diagnosis and risk of prostate cancer progression: data from the cancer of the prostate strategic urologic research endeavor. *Cancer Research* 2011; 71:3889-3895.

54. Lemanne, D. and others, The role of physical activity in cancer prevention, treatment, recovery, and survivorship. *Oncology (Williston Park)* 2013; 27:580-585.

55. Zheng, X. and others, Inhibition of progression of androgen-dependent prostate LNCaP tumors to androgen independence in SCID mice by oral caffeine and voluntary exercise. *Nutrition and Cancer* 2012; 64:1029-1037.

56. Rundqvist, H. and others, Effect of acute exercise on prostate cancer cell growth. *PLoS ONE* 2013 ;8:e67579.

57. Cormie, P. and others, Can supervised exercise prevent treatment toxicity in patients with prostate cancer initiating androgen-deprivation therapy: a randomised controlled trial. *BJU International* 2015; 115:256-266.

58. Mennen-Winchell, L. J. and others, Self-reported exercise and bone mineral density in prostate cancer patients receiving androgen deprivation therapy. *Journal of the American Association of Nurse Practitioners* 2014; 26:40-48.

59. Brown, J. C. and others, The efficacy of exercise in reducing depressive symptoms among cancer survivors: a meta-analysis. *PLoS ONE* 2012; 7:e30955.

60. Zopf, E. M. and others, Effects of a 15-Month Supervised Exercise Program on Physical and Psychological Outcomes in Prostate Cancer Patients Following Prostatectomy: The ProRehab Study. *Integrative Cancer Therapies* 2015; 14:409-18.

61. Geraerts, I. and others, Pelvic floor muscle training for erectile dysfunction and climacturia 1 year after nerve sparing radical prostatectomy: a randomized controlled trial. *International Journal of Impotence Research* 2015; 28;9–13.

62. Bruun, D. M., and others. "All boys and men can play football": a qualitative investigation of recreational football in prostate cancer patients. *Scandinavian Journal of Medicine and Science in Sports* 2014; 24(Suppl.1):113-121.

63. Petticrew, M. and others, Influence of psychological coping on survival and recurrence in people with cancer: systematic review. *British Medical Journal* 2002; 325:1066-1075.

64. Vass, A., Coping with cancer. *British Medical Journal* 2002; 325:1120.

65. Lindberg, P. and others, Breast cancer survivors' recollection of their illness and therapy seven years after enrolment into a randomised controlled clinical trial. *BMC Cancer* 2015; 15:554-566.

66. Watson, M. and others, Influence of psychological response on breast cancer survival: 10-year follow-up of a population-based cohort. *European Journal of Cancer* 2005; 41:1710 – 1714.

67. Soler-Vilá, H. and others, The prognostic role of cancer-specific beliefs among prostate cancer survivors. *Cancer Causes and Control* 2011; 22:251-260.

68. Wang, W. T. and others, Mental adjustment at different phases in breast cancer trajectory: re-examination of factor structure of the Mini-MAC and its correlation with distress. *Psycho-Oncology* 2013; 22:768-74.

69. O'Brien, C. W. and Moorey, S., Outlook and adaptation in advanced cancer: a systematic review. *Psycho-Oncology* 2010; 19:1239-1249.

70. Kim, H. S. and others, Predictors of symptom experience in Korean patients with cancer undergoing chemotherapy. *European Journal of Oncology Nursing* 2015; 19:644-653.

71. Oh, P. J. and Kim, S. H., Effects of a brief psychosocial intervention in patients with cancer receiving adjuvant therapy. *Oncology Nursing Forum* 2010; 37:E98-104.

72. Venetis, M. K. and others, Breast-cancer patients' participation behaviour and coping during presurgical consultations: a pilot study. *Health Communication* 2015; 30:19-25.

73. Tanay, M. A. and others, A time to weep and a time to laugh: humour in the nurse-patient relationship in an adult cancer setting. *Supportive Care in Cancer* 2014; 22:1295-1301.

74. Gawande, A., *The checklist manifesto: how to get things right.* Metropolitan Books of Henry Holt and company LLC: 2009.

75. Haynes, A. B. and others, A surgical safety checklist to reduce morbidity and mortality in a global population. *The New England Journal of Medicine* 2009; 360:491-499.

76. Lynch, J. J., *The broken heart: the medical consequences of loneliness.* Basic Books, 1977.

77. Kaplan, R. M. and Kronick, R. G., Marital status and longevity in the United States population. *Journal of Epidemiology and Community Health* 2006; 60:760-65.

78. Manzoli, L. and others, Marital status and mortality in the elderly: a systematic review and meta-analysis. *Social Science and Medicine* 2007; 64:77-94.

79. Scafato, E. and others, Marital and cohabitation status as predictors of mortality: a 10-year follow-up of an Italian elderly cohort. *Social Science & Medicine* 2008; 67:1456-1464.

80. Pillay, B. and others, Psychosocial factors predicting survival after allogeneic stem cell transplant. *Supportive Care in Cancer* 2014; 22:2547-2555.

81. Tyson, M. D. and others, Marital status and prostate cancer outcomes. *Canadian Journal of Urology* 2013;20:6702-6706.

82. Pinquart M, Duberstein PR. Associations of social networks with cancer mortality: a meta-analysis. *Critical Reviews in Oncology-Hematology* 2010; 75:122-137.

83. Beasley, J. M. and others, Social networks and survival after breast cancer diagnosis. *Journal of Cancer Survivorship* 2010; 4:372-380.

84. Rottenberg, Y. and others, Prediagnostic self-assessed health and extent of social networks predict survival in older individuals with cancer: a population based cohort study. *Journal of Geriatric Oncology* 2014; 5:400-407.

85. Mols, F. and others, Quality of life among long-term breast cancer survivors: a systematic review. *European Journal of Cancer* 2005; 41:2613–2619.

86. Goodwin, L. and others, I've had a good life, what's left is a bonus: factor analysis of the mental adjustment to cancer scale in a palliative care population. *Palliative Medicine* 2014; 28:243-255.

87. Zucca, A. C. and others, Life is precious and I'm making the best of it: coping strategies of long-term cancer survivors. *Psycho-Oncology* 2010; 19:1268-1276.

88. Berglund, A. and others, Differences according to socioeconomic status in the management and mortality in men with high risk prostate cancer. *European Journal of Cancer* 2012; 48:75-84.

89. Chu, D. I. and others, Effect of race and socioeconomic status on surgical margins and biochemical outcomes in an equal-access health care setting: results from the Shared Equal Access Regional Cancer Hospital (SEARCH) database. *Cancer* 2012; 118:4999-5007.

90. Shafique, K. and Morrison, K., Socio-economic inequalities in survival of patients with prostate cancer: role of age and Gleason grade at diagnosis. *PLoS ONE* 2013; 8:e56184.

91. Rayford, W., Managing the low-socioeconomic-status prostate cancer patient. *Journal of the National Medical Association* 2006; 98:521-530.

92. Bell, A., "I think about Oprah": social class differences in sources of health information. *Qualitative Health Research* 2014; 24:506-516.

93. Sivarajan, G. and others, Ten-year outcomes of sexual function after radical prostatectomy: results of a prospective longitudinal study. *European Urology* 2014; 65:58-65.

94. Schover, L. R. and others, Defining sexual outcomes after treatment for localised prostate carcinoma. *Cancer* 2002; 95:1773-1785.

95. Mulhall, J. P., Defining and reporting erectile function outcomes after radical prostatectomy: challenges and misconceptions. *Journal of Urology* 2009; 181:462-471.

96. Barnas, J. L. and others, The prevalence and nature of orgasmic dysfunction after radical prostatectomy. *BJU International* 2004; 94:603-605.

97. Tran, S. N. and others, Prospective evaluation of early postoperative male and female sexual function after radical prostatectomy with erectile nerves preservation. *International Journal of Impotence Research* 2015; 27:69-74.

98. Lee, T. K. and others, Impact of prostate cancer treatment on the sexual quality of life for Men-Who-Have-Sex-with-Men. *Journal of Sexual Medicine* 2015; 12:2378-2386.

99. Degauqier, C. and others, Impact of aging on sexuality. *Revue Medicale de Bruxelles* 2012; 33:153-163.

100. *The Royal College of Pathologists.* Standards and datasets for reporting cancers. Dataset for histopathology reports for prostatic carcinoma. June 2016.

101. Rees, J. and others, Diagnosis and treatment of chronic bacterial prostatitis and chronic prostatitis/chronic pelvic pain syndrome: a consensus guideline. *BJU International* 2015; 116:509-525.

102. Stancik, I. and others, Effect of NIH-IV prostatitis on free and free-to-total PSA. European Urology 2004; 46:760-764.

103. Loeb, S. and Sandhu, J. S., Use of empiric antibiotics in the setting of an increased prostate specific antigen. *Journal of Urology* 2011; 186:17-19.

104. Algra. A. M. and Rothwell, P.M., Effects of regular aspirin on long-term cancer incidence and metastasis: a systematic comparison of evidence from observational studies versus randomised trials. *Lancet Oncology* 2012; 13:518-527.
105. Bibbins-Domingo, K., on behalf of the U.S. Preventive Services Task Force. Aspirin Use for the Primary Prevention of Cardiovascular Disease and Colorectal Cancer: U.S. Preventive Services Task Force Recommendation Statement. *Annals of Internal Medicine* 2016; 164:836-845.
106. Elwood, P. C. and others. Aspirin in the Treatment of Cancer: Reductions in Metastatic Spread and in Mortality: A Systematic Review and Meta-Analyses of Published Studies. *PLoS ONE* 2016; 11:e0152402.
107. Farwell, W. R. and others. Statins and prostate cancer diagnosis and grade in a veterans population. *Journal of the National Cancer Institute* 2011; 103:885-892.
108. Harshman, L. C. and others, Statin use at the time of initiation of androgen deprivation therapy and time to progression in patients with hormone-sensitive prostate cancer. *JAMA Oncology* 2015; 1:495-504.
109. Hong, S. K. and others, Prognostic significance of undetectable ultrasensitive prostate-specific antigen nadir after radical prosta-tectomy. *Urology* 2010; 76:723-727.
110. Karlin, J. D. and others, Identifying appropriate patients for early salvage radiotherapy after prostatectomy. *Journal of Urology* 2013; 190:1410-1415.
111. O'Neill, R. F. and others, A randomised controlled trial to evalu-ate the efficacy of a 6-month dietary and physical activity inter-vention for patients receiving androgen deprivation therapy for prostate cancer. *Journal of Cancer Survivorship* 2015; 9:431-440.
112. Crook, J. M. and others, Intermittent androgen suppression for rising PSA Level after radiotherapy. *New England Journal of Medicine* 2012; 367:895-903.
113. Hussain, M. and others, Intermittent versus continuous andro-gen deprivation in prostate cancer. *New England Journal of Medicine* 2013; 368:1314-1325.
114. Klotz, L., Intermittent androgen deprivation therapy: clarity from confusion. *European Urology* 2013; 64:731-733.

115. Magnan, S. and others, Intermittent vs continuous androgen deprivation therapy for prostate cancer: a systematic review and meta-analysis. *JAMA Oncology* 2015; 1:1261-1269.

116. Hershman, D. L. and others, Adverse health events following intermittent and continuous androgen deprivation in patients with metastatic prostate cancer. *JAMA Oncology* 2016; 2:453-461.

117. Liede, A. and others, International survey of androgen deprivation therapy (ADT) for non-metastatic prostate cancer in 19 countries. *ESMO Open* 2016; 1:e000040.

118. Schweizer, M. T. and others, Bipolar Androgen Therapy for men with androgen ablation naïve prostate cancer: results from the phase II BATMAN study. *Prostate* 2016; 76:1218-1226.

119. Kiciński, M. and others. An epidemiological reappraisal of the familial aggregation of prostate cancer: a meta-analysis. *PLoS ONE* 2011; 6: e27130.

120. Chen, Y. C. and others, Family history of prostate and breast cancer and the risk of prostate cancer in the PSA era. *Prostate* 2008; 68:1582-91.

Lightning Source UK Ltd.
Milton Keynes UK
UKOW06f0707280517

302152UK00011B/62/P